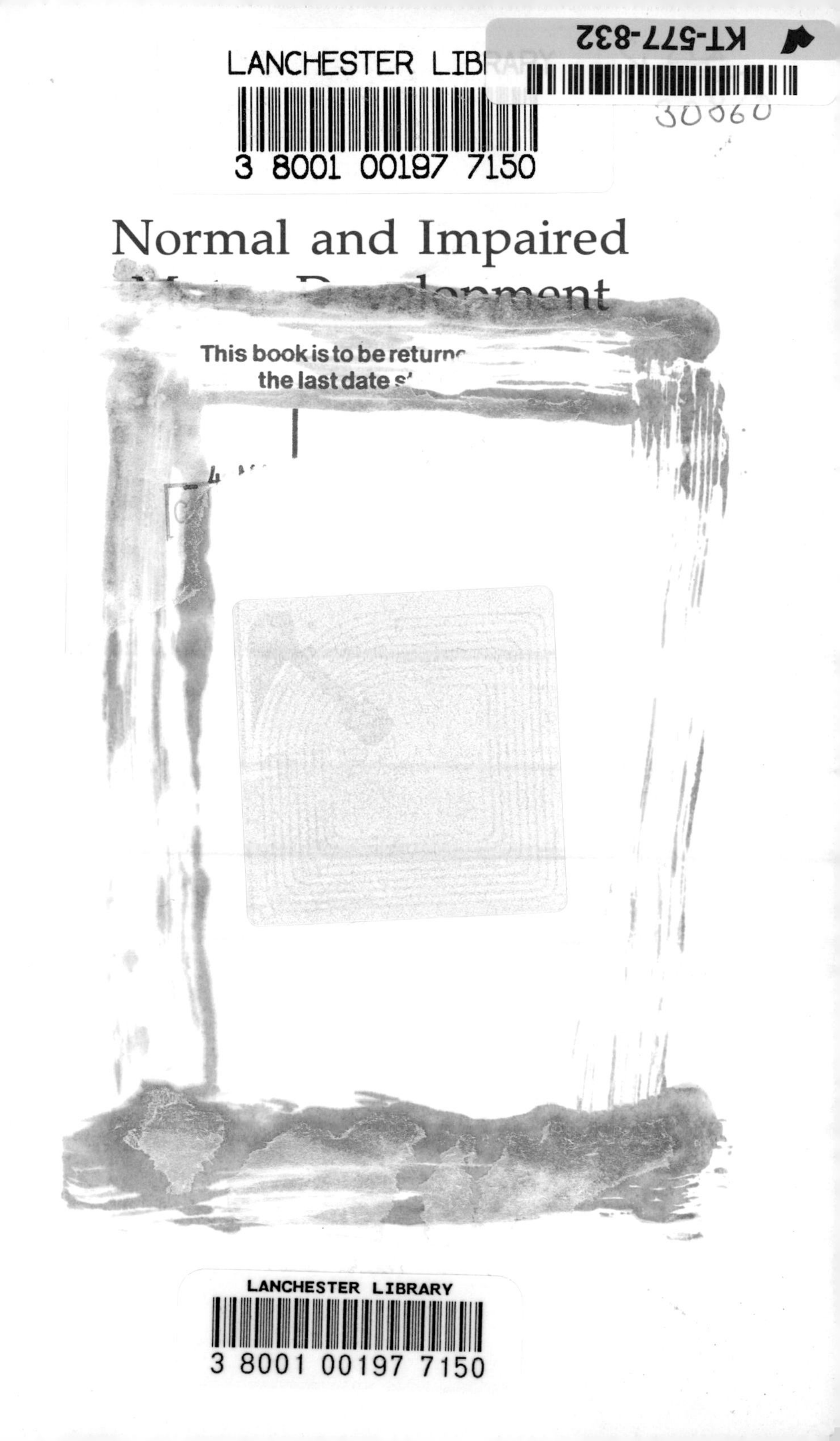
LANCHESTER LIBRARY
3 8001 00197 7150
Normal and Impaired
This book is to be return
the last date
LANCHESTER LIBRARY
3 8001 00197 7150

Normal and Impaired Motor Development

Theory into Practice

Carolyn O'Brien

Lecturer at the School of Human Movement Studies,
Queensland University of Technology, Australia

and

Alan Hayes

Associate Professor at the Fred and Eleanor Schonell
Special Education Research Centre,
University of Queensland, Australia

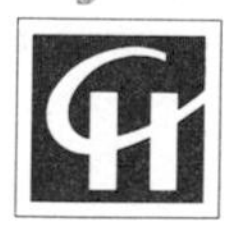

CHAPMAN & HALL

London · Glasgow · Weinheim · New York · Tokyo · Melbourne · Madras

Published by Chapman & Hall, 2–6 Boundary Row, London SE1 8HN, UK

Chapman & Hall, 2–6 Boundary Row, London SE1 8HN, UK

Blackie Academic & Professional, Wester Cleddens Road, Bishopbriggs, Glasgow G64 2NZ, UK

Chapman & Hall GmbH, Pappelallee 3, 69469 Weinheim, Germany

Chapman & Hall USA, One Penn Plaza, 41st Floor, New York NY 10119, USA

Chapman & Hall Japan, ITP-Japan, Kyowa Building, 3F, 2-2-1 Hirakawacho, Chiyoda-ku, Tokyo 102, Japan

Chapman & Hall Australia, Thomas Nelson Australia, 102 Dodds Street, South Melbourne, Victoria 3205, Australia

Chapman & Hall India, R. Seshadri, 32 Second Main Road, CIT East, Madras 600 035, India

---

Distributed in the USA and Canada by Singular Publishing Group Inc., 4284 41st Street, San Diego, California 92105

First edition 1995

Typeset in 10/12pt Palatino by Mews Photosetting, Beckenham, Kent
Printed in Great Britain by St Edmundsbury Press, Bury St Edmunds

ISBN 0 412 47890 0 1 56593 148 3 (USA)

A catalogue record for this book is available from the British Library

Library of Congress Catalog Card Number: 94-68790

∞ Printed on permanent acid-free text paper, manufactured in accordance with ANSI/NISO Z39.48–1992 and ANSI/NISO Z39.48–1984 (Permanence of Paper).

Contents

Acknowledgements

As with most books, the production of this volume has been facilitated and enriched by the support, encouragement and contributions of many people. First, and foremost, we must gratefully acknowledge the assistance of the many children who participated in the research that has culminated in this work. To them, and their families, we say without your willing assistance there would have been no book. Second, we must express our appreciation of the encouragement and skilled editorial involvement of Catherine Walker and Lisa Fraley, of Chapman & Hall, who together with the comments of two anonymous reviewers, have smoothed the path in so many ways. Finally, without the encouragement, understanding and support of our families we would have found the long hours of drafting, re-drafting and editorial polishing very difficult to endure. This book is dedicated to Ralph and Karen and our children Rosemary, Caitlin, Eris, and Sarah. Thanks does not capture the depth of our appreciation of your support.

Introduction

The main aim of this book is to provide a framework for studying normal and impaired motor development. Using this framework, guidelines are described for the development of intervention programmes for motor impaired children. Developmental progression in movement behaviour is a central organizing theme. The authors are of the opinion that it is only by studying movement against the backdrop of normal development, that delayed or different movement behaviour can be understood (see Chapters 1 and 2 for the conceptual framework from which motor development is examined). Research literature and a series of original studies are also reported. The studies explored the developmental progressions of motor impaired children, focusing particularly on children who are clumsy, intellectually disabled or with Down syndrome. These three groups were chosen because they were considered to have problems that involve aspects of sensory-neurological, perceptual-integrative and motor-learning control dysfunction which contribute to their particular motor impairments.

As a basis for intervention, the authors describe a multidimensional assessment model, examining motor performance, fundamental movement patterns and interlimb coordination. These three aspects have been chosen for particular attention for the following reasons. Motor performance scores are commonly used to provide an initial indication of each child's motor development (Chapter 3). These tests bear some similarities to intelligence tests as they are norm-referenced, usually by age. The scores they provide are believed to reflect maturational and physical development.

Performance on these tests is influenced by sensory-neurological, perceptual-integrative and motor learning-control processes and the amount of practice or experience a child has had in a specific motor skill.

By only testing motor performance, however, insufficient information is available to design programmes to address the specific movement problems of individual children. For example, the motor performance scores do not give any indication as to why children performed below the average level for their age. Furthermore, although two children might obtain a similar score for motor performance, observation revealed that the quality and pattern of their basic movements differed. It was suspected that there were two reasons for these observed differences. In some cases it appeared that children showed less maturity in their movement patterns while, in others, the children gave some indications of problems in their control of movement.

The second area within the multidimensional assessment model is evaluation of fundamental movement patterns. A new assessment device, the Fundamental Movement Pattern Profiles (FMPP) was developed to provide a qualitative, descriptive, observational measure. The profiles in this book were derived from descriptions of movement patterns provided by previous researchers and were developed and tested by the authors, first on normally developing children, then on groups of motor impaired children (Chapters 4 and 5).

The third area which was assessed was cognitive control of movement. This led to experimentation with an interlimb coordination task. Such a task is another means of detecting the effect of dysfunction in motor control processes and response organization in motor impaired children. Results of research into interlimb bimanual coordination of motor impaired children are reported in Chapter 6.

To assist your use of this book the contents comprise relevant literature reviews on motor development in normally developing and motor impaired children; motor performance; fundamental movement patterns; motor control and a discussion of the results from studies to determine whether motor impaired children (specifically, children who are clumsy, intellectually disabled or have Down syndrome) are developmentally delayed or different in their motor behaviour. This material is organized as follows.

Chapter 1: Overview of Motor Development first discusses the progression of normal movement behaviour. It then introduces the reader to a neurobehavioural framework incorporating the concepts of sensory-neurological, perceptual-integrative and motor learning-control processes that affect movement behaviour. In subsequent chapters, this framework is also used to examine the motor development of children who are clumsy, intellectually disabled or have Down syndrome.

Chapter 2: Motor Development in Movement Impaired Children reviews the literature on motor differences between normally developing, clumsy, intellectually disabled and children with Down syndrome. These differences in motor development are then discussed under the headings of sensory-neurological, perceptual-integrative and motor learning-control processes.

Chapter 3: Motor Performance examines factors that affect motor performance in children who are normally developing, clumsy, intellectually disabled and with Down syndrome children and reports on a study, by the authors, conducted to determine differences between normally developing and motor impaired children.

Chapter 4: Fundamental Movement Patterns comprises a literature review on the normal developmental progression of children in walking, running, jumping, throwing and catching. It also has pictorial sequences of developmental progression in these fundamental movement patterns.

Chapter 5: Sequences of Fundamental Movement Patterns examines methodological and research issues reported in the literature that are relevant to the development of fundamental movement pattern sequences. These sequences were used to examine the developmental progression of the fundamental movements patterns of clumsy, intellectually disabled and children with Down syndrome.

Chapter 6: Motor Control reviews relevant literature in motor control in adults and children with a special section reviewing the motor control of children with Down syndrome. Interlimb tasks are also reviewed in adults and children and the discussion is illustrated with data from a study of bimanual interlimb control. The study explored limb coordination differences among normally developing, clumsy, intellectually disabled and children with Down syndrome.

Chapter 7: Summary, Implications and Conclusions from the Present Studies: Recommendations for Physical Activity Programmes As well as the summary and conclusions, this chapter contains guidelines for the design of intervention programmes as well as examples of activities for use with motor impaired children. The activities are presented under the headings, sensory–motor, perceptual–motor and cognitive–motor to suit children from basic, intermediate and advanced levels of motor development.

1

Overview of motor development

This chapter describes a framework for underlying processes that occur in the acquisition of skilled movements. An understanding of typical movement behaviour provides the basis for evaluating delay or difference in motor development. To assist in this understanding, a hierarchical progression of motor behaviour in children will be discussed, followed by an examination of sensory-neurological, integrative-perceptual and motor learning-control processes which are considered to influence normal developmental changes in motor behaviour.

OVERVIEW

Throughout their development children undergo surprisingly rapid changes in their movement skills. The often jerky, inefficient movements of the infant or the older clumsy child, change to the more efficient, smooth attempts of older children (Connolly, 1980). These observable differences between infancy and childhood in movement behaviour, according to some theorists, are due both to maturation and learning, resulting in more efficient motor control and response organization in older children (Charlton, 1992; Clark and Whitall, 1989). Implicit in this assumption is that to understand the development of skilled movement in young children, it is necessary to study the changes which occur as children become increasingly competent in these skills. Such an approach expands the traditional description of changes which occur with age, in the performance of movement patterns, such as sitting or climbing.

It also seeks to understand the development of underlying processes which may be related to these changes (Keogh, 1977; Keogh and Sugden, 1985).

MOTOR DEVELOPMENT

Motor development can be thought of as a process that begins before birth and continues throughout adult life. Early movement sequences are considered to be biologically determined because they are dependent on physiological and neurological maturation (Ames and Ilg, 1964, 1966). Skilled movements, in contrast, are dependent on the combination of maturation, practice and learning (Malina, 1984; O'Brien, 1994; Thomas, 1984).

It was generally accepted by earlier developmental researchers that the steady improvement in children's motor skills was due to maturation and experience (Ames and Ilg, 1964; Gesell, 1973). In normal development children become able to perform more complex movements. Further, there is similarity in the way in which children achieve new motor skills. On the basis of the broad similarity in the progression of movement behaviour, it has been argued that all children progress through a relatively similar sequence of development, even though the rate of progression may vary (McGraw, 1966; Shirley, 1931). It has been demonstrated, however, that children's development is influenced by the interaction of internal and external factors and it is this interaction that helps to explain why there are individual differences in children's development and behaviour (Fischer and Farrar, 1988).

Some of the internal factors that contribute to differences in the rate of motor development in children include growth and biological maturation, increase in cognitive capacity, and personality and motivation. For example, physical changes in bones, muscles and the cardiovascular system give greater body strength, endurance and mechanical advantage when performing sport skills (Malina, 1984; Newell, 1984). Changes in neural structure and brain tissue enable faster transmission of neural impulses and coding of movement information (Thomas, 1984; Touwen, 1976). These changes result in a faster motor response together with the ability to perform more complex movements. In addition, an improvement in cognitive capacity in children as they mature allows them to direct their attention to relevant sources of movement information which in turn, facilitates the learning of more complex movements and skills (Schmidt, 1988; Thomas, 1984).

Personality and motivation of children are also very important because if they feel competent about their skills and enjoy experimentation, they will experience a wider variety of movements than other children. Conversely, overanxious children and those who feel incompetent may withdraw from new situations and so fall further behind their peers in movement skills.

Other important factors are nutrition, health and fitness. Malnourished, unhealthy or unfit children are often deprived of a variety of movement experiences as they tire easily. It has been shown in an extensive multidisciplinary study, for example, that many children identified in Brisbane, Australia by their teachers as the most reluctant to participate in physical activity and sport in primary schools, had neurological deficits such as low muscle tone, visual tracking problems or were asthmatics. As a group, the non-participating children also were very unfit and most were overweight (O'Brien *et al.*, 1993).

External, environmental factors which affect motor development include the amount of stimulation children receive. The amount of movement stimulation children receive will either enhance or delay their motor development, so in some children their apparent motor delay is due to lack of experience, not to any biological factors. Another important environmental factor is the amount of time young children play and older children spend in games, sport, dance and gymnastics. These activities ensure that they are practising movement skills, which leads to greater body awareness and movement control.

In order to enhance motor development, people who care for, or work with, children should be aware of the importance of both sets of factors. It also means that individual differences in motor development will increase with age, partly because of differences in children's personality, their biological bases of movement and environmental experiences.

Although biological and environmental factors make an important contribution to children's individual differences in movement behaviour, in the remainder of this chapter the theoretical framework on aspects of motor development will be discussed. First, by tracing the observable progression of movement behaviours, then by sketching the underlying processes which affect normal motor development. Finally, a perspective emphasizing three phases of motor development will be outlined and from this perspective suitable guidelines and activities for developmental motor intervention will be examined.

PROGRESSION OF OBSERVABLE MOVEMENT BEHAVIOURS

Observable developmental changes in movement behaviour can be ordered into a hierarchy, progressing from relatively simple movement to complex skills (Table 1.1). The assumption of a hierarchy of movement behaviour is that the developmental sequence starts with reflexes which are movement responses that the infant cannot control and progresses to highly skilled movements which are dependent on motor learning and control factors. Children need normal sensory and neurological development as the basis for the integration and perception of movement information, which then enables them to develop awareness and control of their movements. Extensive learning and practice in specific movement situations is necessary for the acquisition of complex skills.

Table 1.1 Progression of movement behaviours

1. *Reflexes* are neurally predefined movements, triggered by a stimulus such as touch, sound, or a movement stimulus to parts of the body, examples include sucking, grasping and postural reflexes.
2. *Movement patterns based on reflex actions* are automatic patterns incorporated into a movement sequence such as those used in early attempts at walking and fine motor manual skills.
3. *Between (intertask) skill movement sequences* are a transition phase between early reflex-based movements and cognitively controlled movements, for example, by using these movements together with developmental milestones the child might change postures by rolling from the back to the stomach, to sitting then standing, in order to attain an upright posture.
4. *Within (intratask) skill movement sequences* occur when the child acquires and refines movements within clearly defined skills such as walking, running, jumping, catching and throwing.
5. *Complex movement skills* are learnt movement sequences such as those used in handwriting, ballet, athletics, gymnastics, swimming and tennis.

Each of the defined progressions in movement behaviour will now be discussed.

Reflex movements

A reflex movement occurs when a child makes a stereotyped movement response to a stimulus without being able to control that response (Bobath, 1985; Fiorentino, 1974). Reflex movements begin when the fetus is about 2 cm in length (Touwen, 1976; Wolf, 1986). Some of these prenatal reflex movements consist of flexion and extension of all the limbs, similar to the steroetyped limb movements of the newborn baby (Thelen, 1983). In newborn babies, reflexes are important for their survival. As babies grow reflexes help develop muscular strength, they allow children to interact with their environment and according to some researchers, they develop units of movements which are incorporated into skilled movements used later in life (Easton, 1977; Eliasson, Gordon and Forssberg, 1991; Holt, 1975).

Reflexes in newborn babies can be thought of as inbuilt survival mechanisms that enable them to suck, swallow, sneeze, turn their heads, support their own weight by hanging onto a rod, and make alternate stepping and swimming movements. Reflex movements related to the position of the head also result in changes occurring in muscle tension in different parts of the body and so affect limb and body position. In the newborn when the head is tipped forward, for example, the limbs are flexed and moved in towards the body. In contrast, when the head is tipped backwards the limbs are extended and moved out and away from the body. These are some of the earliest whole body reflexes which help to maintain muscle tone and postural stability throughout life.

In the process of normal maturation the primitive reflexes are replaced by midbrain reflexes. Even more mature body and postural reflexes are needed throughout life to adjust a person's head, trunk and limbs, automatically, in order to maintain balance (Bobath, 1985, Roberton, 1984; Rochat, 1992). In addition to the reflex actions already described, those such as the early grasp reflexes that are present in newborn children elicit predetermined finger movements that will be incorporated into the many more advanced skills (Pretchl, 1986).

Some of these skills include the ability to grasp, manipulate and release objects, that give us the necessary movement patterns to learn fine motor skills such as handwriting, typing and sewing (O'Brien and Ziviani, 1991).

Movements based on reflex actions

As has already been mentioned, movements resulting from reflexes that control large and small body movements are incorporated as units of movement into some of the early walking and grasping actions. The walking reflex is a good example. It occurs when babies from about four to twelve weeks of age are held up under the armpits, so that their legs are extended and although their feet are in contact with the ground they are only taking some of their body weight. In this position they perform alternate stepping actions. It has been shown that practice of the walking reflex results in incorporation of this pattern into babies' movement repertoires, so they walk at an earlier age than those who have not regularly practised this reflex (Zelazo, 1983). Similarly, it has been demonstrated that placing visually attractive objects within their reach results in the appearance of visually guided reaching for objects earlier than babies who were not provided with stimulating visual environments (White, 1970).

It appears then that some reflex patterns and early motor responses are directly incorporated into voluntarily controlled units of movement, that have been named synergies (Lee, 1984), or coordinative structures (Easton, 1977) or subroutines (Connolly, 1980). This contradicts Gesell (1973), who was of the opinion that early reflexes, such as the moro, asymmetrical and symmetrical tonic neck reflexes, must be inhibited in the central nervous system before voluntary control of movement was possible. He argued that when these reflexes dominate movement behaviour, as they do in severely cerebral palsied children, they interfere with advanced voluntary control of movement (Bobath, 1985; Yokachi *et al.*, 1993).

The postural reflexes are another important group of reflexes that are considered necessary for normal motor development. Many of them are used and modified to assist in the maintenance of postural stability throughout life (Ayres, 1982; Bobath, 1985; Fiorentino, 1974; Woollacott, Shumway-Cook and

Williams, 1989). Contrary to Gesell's opinions, it would appear, then, that these automated units of movement form the basic building blocks of many complex and skilled movements.

Between-task (intertask) movement sequences

These movements consist of rotation and weight transference, which enable children to link some of the already acquired developmental milestones such as sitting and standing into movement sequences that assist them in exploring their environment. Between-task movement sequences are a very important transition from reflex movements to more complex skills. If children do not have these rotational and weight transference movements in their repertoire they are unable to continue progressing normally in their motor development. Children with Down syndrome, for instance, often learn to maintain their balance while sitting by having their legs very wide apart (Block, 1991; Lydic and Steele, 1979). This posture enables them to sit, but if it persists it hinders rotational movements, so inhibiting the normal progression from this position of rotating sideways and transferring the weight onto all four limbs to achieve a crawling position and vice versa.

An example of an intertask sequence is demonstrated by children when they try to walk. They often proceed from the sitting position to the crawling position to a semi-upright stance with both hands and feet on the floor, to holding onto and cruising around furniture, to a tentative stance on the feet and finally to the first unsteady walking steps (Shirley, 1931). Another example is the fine motor sequence of early reach, grasp and release used by children when they first start manipulating objects (O'Brien and Ziviani, 1991).

The attainment of between-task movement sequences is an indication that children's movement skills are developing normally. These movement sequences, however, are only part of the picture of motor development. The within-task movement sequences (discussed in the next section) are another important aspect of motor skill development.

Within-task (intratask) movement sequences

The sequence of changes within each of the fundamental movement skills of walking, running, jumping, catching and throwing are called within-task (intratask) movement sequences. These changes, which are partly due to increased maturation and experience, have been shown to be similar in the majority of children, in regard to increased control of dynamic balance, limb and body movements.

Once children have acquired more advanced levels of fundamental movement patterns for locomotion and manipulation they have greater control over their physical environment. Research on the progressive refinement of the fundamental movement patterns (Chapter 4) provides much information about the developmental status of children, as well as providing clues into the important sensory, neurological, integrative, perceptual, motor learning and control processes that children are undergoing.

Complex movement skills

Skilled movements are characterized by spatial and temporal accuracy in performing a movement task. They can be modified according to changes in physical and environmental demands and different movements can be produced to solve new movement tasks (Glencross, 1980; Keogh and Sugden, 1985). Processes which affect the observable changes in movement control can be conceptualized as being due to the interaction between control processes underlying the progression through the movement hierarchy.

Changes in young children's early movement patterns and developmental milestones, for example, may be considered as predominantly due to sensory and neurological processes. Movements which become more refined with environmental interaction and practice are due more to integrative, perceptual, motor learning and control processes. More advanced motor learning and control of movement, together with a greater knowledge base and repertoire of learned movement patterns, enable children to acquire the complex skills needed for participation in everyday activities and games (e.g. Glencross, 1980; Newell, 1985; van Wierington, 1986).

From this brief overview of the progression of movement behaviour, it is apparent that hierarchical changes in movement can be conceptualized as progressing from simpler to more complex movements. Implicit in this notion is that simpler movement behaviours are more representative of more basic processes, whereas complex movements require greater cognitive motor control. According to this neurobehavioural perspective, sensory and neurological processes will affect children's knowledge and early awareness of their bodies and their movements. Integrative, perceptual, motor learning and control processes increase the potential quality and range of their movement skills (Keogh and Sugden, 1985)

A NEUROBEHAVIOURAL PERSPECTIVE ON MOVEMENT

A neurobehavioural perspective has been adopted in this book to identify and discuss some of the processes that influence observable maturational and learning related changes in children's movement behaviour. The processes which comprise the underlying basis of movement are outlined in Table 1.2 and then discussed in more detail in the next section.

Sensory-neurological processes (basic processes)

Use of sensory systems

Sensory systems are usually classified as exteroceptive receptors that receive information from the external envrionment and proprioceptive receptors that receive internal bodily stimuli from structures, for example, within the inner ear (vestibular system) and within the muscles and joints (kinaesthetic system). Both types of systems enable us to feel and respond to sensations from our external and internal environments. Knowledge of the environment is gained from touch, taste, sound and movement, whereas internal information from the vestibular and kinaesthetic system provides information vital for movement control. As the roles of the vestibular and kinaesthetic systems appear to be less well known, they will now be described in more detail.

Table 1.2 Neurobehavioural processes in motor development

Sensory-neurological processes (basic processes)

These processes represent the automatic basis of all movements. Children may still be able to acquire complex movements even though they may have dysfunction in these basic areas, but the quality and control of their movements will not be of the same standard as people who have well developed sensory-neurological processes. Two of these basic processes are:

Use of sensory systems: visual, auditory, tactile, vestibular and kinaesthetic systems provide the initial sensory information which is necessary for development of body and movement awareness.

Maintenance of muscle tone: provides the amount of tension around the joints which enables some of the body segments to maintain stability while other segments move; also, sufficient muscle tone is essential for maintenance of postural stability.

Integrative-perceptual processes (intermediate processes)

These processes involve the integration of early movements with sensory information from the visual, vestibular and kinaesethetic sensory systems; these are the three most important sensory systems for movement production. Such processes underlie perceptual awareness and control of the body, additionally, they form the framework for the development of more complex movements. Some of the important processes are:

Sensory integration and body perception: the ability to synthesize visual, auditory, tactile, vestibular and kinaesthetic information relevant to the production of movement, so enabling children to acquire body, visual–spatial and spatial awareness, to control the limbs and to develop hand–eye and foot–eye coordination.

Maintenance of postural stability: the ability to maintain functional posture is dependent on adequate muscle tone, postural reflexes and the ability to integrate visual, sensory and peceptual information.

Motor learning-control processes (advanced processes)

These processes enable greater ability to control and learn movements and a consequent increased ability (a) to perform complex movements, (b) to respond effectively to external criteria, (c) to execute smoother more fluent and better timed movements and (d) to generate new and novel movements to achieve predetermined goals. These processes are necessary for improvement in limb and hand–eye coordination and in the acquisition of a wide range of movement skills, they include:

Motor learning: which refers to increased levels of complexity of information processing and the ability to remember complex movement sequences.

Motor control: which results in improved ability to control an ongoing motor response.

The vestibular system

Together with touch, the vestibular system is one of the sensory systems that develops earliest. This system responds to movement of the head and in so doing provides us with information about body position and motion in relation to ourselves and to the external environment. Such information is essential as the majority of motor skills depend on the maintenance of postural stability.

The sensory organs responsible for vestibular information are located within the labyrinth of the inner ear. Major information is derived from the three semicircular canals in the inner ear. These canals are orientated horizontally, vertically and obliquely. They are filled with fluid and they also contain 'hair-like' nerve endings which respond to the movement of the fluid within the semicircular canals due to changes in direction and rotational movements. Information from the vestibular system is important in the maintenance of balance, but another important aspect is its contribution to visual fixation and maintenance of muscle tone (Gabbard, 1992; Schmidt, 1988).

Children with vestibular system dysfunction or delay are often fearful of heights and exhibit poor spatial perception. Generally, they do not like activities which involve them moving off the ground. Many children who have low vestibular awareness seek fast movements or spinning activities and appear to have little awareness of danger (O'Brien,1991).

The kinaesthetic system

This provides the person with movement information derived from a group of sensory receptors. Some of the important receptors are: the Golgi tendon organs, located at the musculotendinous junction, that respond to tension in the muscles; the muscle spindle receptors that respond to stretch of the fibres; and the joint receptors that respond to pressure, position and range of movement (Gabbard, 1992; Lazlo and Bairstow, 1985; Schmidt, 1988). The kinaesthetic system is important because it provides information about bodily movement without reference to the external receptors of vision and audition. Such information is essential for the maintenance of an appropriate posture and for the control of muscle tone and the coding of movement information in memory, which assists the learning of skilled movements.

Children who have developmental delay or dysfunction in their kinaesthetic system usually have low body awareness in comparison with their normally developing peers. If they have low muscle tone they usually appear to be 'floppy' or weak, or else they compensate for low tone and poor body awareness by tensing their muscles and often hyperextending their joints to provide them with increased kinaesthetic information. Both groups of children have lessened body awareness, which can be observed, for example, when they are asked to imitate another person's movements (O'Brien, 1991).

Maintenance of muscle tone

Normal movements are partially dependent on normal muscle tone. Muscle tone refers to the amount of tension in the resting muscle and is due largely to the mechanical properties of the Golgi tendon organs, muscle spindles and muscle fibres (Schmidt, 1988; Walsh, 1992). It is assessed by the excitability of the stretch reflex, that is, the amount of resistance that can be applied to a contracted muscle or muscle group, and the presence or absence of a complete range of motion around a joint (Cameron-Tucker, 1983; Daniels and Worthingham, 1980). The amount of muscle tone a person has is due to many factors including the elastic property of tendons and muscle fibres and the amount of motor unit activity which is dependent on the excitability of the nervous system (Wyke, 1976).

In behavioural terms low muscle tone is associated with low body awareness, because kinaesthetic input is affected, whereas high tone is often associated with rigidity of the muscles (Levitt, 1979). Children with Down syndrome characteristically have low muscle tone, which probably contributes to their poor body awareness and their difficulty in maintaining normal postural stability (Davis and Kelso, 1982; Shepherd, 1980). In contrast, children with spasticity have very high muscle tone in affected limbs which causes contractures around the joints in these limbs and abnormal gait patterns (Bobath, 1985; Leonard, Hirschfeld and Forssberg, 1991).

Integrative-Perceptual Processes (intermediate processes)

Sensory integration and perception

Sensory integration is dependent on three processes: the recognition of sensory information; identification that a stimulus may come from the same source, even when it is presented in different modalities; and cross-modal transfer, which is the ability to transfer sensory stimuli from one sensory modality to another, in order to perform complex tasks such as maintaining postural stability (Gabbard, 1992; Jones, 1981). Developmental changes in children's movement behaviour, especially in regard to knowledge about their bodies, are partly dependent on the ability to integrate and interpret sensory information based on past experiences. It has already been mentioned that the information for movement is derived from visual, auditory, tactile, vestibular and kinaesthetic systems. Integration of sensory information is important because it enables children to develop a conscious perception about their bodies and their movements.

Visual perception, for example, is an important process in regard to development of movement behaviour. Visual acuity, spatial orientation and figure perception operate at an adult level before 12 years of age. Other aspects of visual–motor coordination are more complex and develop later (Gabbard, 1992).

Kinaesthetic perception is fundamental to an awareness of the body and its movements. This awareness is demonstrated behaviourally when children show they know that the body has two sides (left and right), that limbs can be coordinated in different patterns (interlimb coordination) and the body can be moved in different directions such as up, down, sideways, forwards and backwards. Children also develop spatial awareness in relation to their own bodies and to external objects (Gabbard, 1992).

As children become more competent in visual and kinaesthetic perceptual processes they are able to make increasingly more accurate judgements about speed and direction of moving objects and they are able to perform more complex movements. In this way normal infants are able to develop more mature motor patterns and movement behaviours

(Lazlo and Bairstow, 1982). Integration of kinaesthetic and visual information is essential to the maintenance of postural stability (Woollacott, Shumway-Cook and Williams, 1989).

Maintenance of postural stability

Maintenance of postural stability is a good example of an integrative process that is an important component of performing many motor skills (Burton and Davis, 1992). It is dependent on a complex interaction between sensory and motor systems, the integration of sensory information, maturation of normal postural reflexes and regulation of normal muscle tone (Bobath, 1985; Horak *et al.*, 1988; Thelen, 1983). The importance of sensory information for the maintenance of postural stability is demonstrated by the fact that visual and vestibular input are seen as alternate sensory inputs and that kinaesethetic information derived from movement at the ankle joint, is linked with visual and vestibular information to determine postural sway (Nashner, 1976; Woolacott, Shumway-Cook and Williams, 1989).

Some of the important postural reflexes necessary for the maintenance of postural stability are the tonic neck and labyrinthine reflexes that are activated by position and movement of the head. As the importance of these reflexes diminishes, receptors in the neck muscle and ankle joints provide the information required to maintain postural stability (Abrahams, 1982). The role of normal postural reflexes in development of postural stability was demonstrated by a study of mildly to moderately intellectually disabled children. This study showed that although these children had normal muscle tone they were not progressing to more mature postural milestones because they had delayed postural reflexes (Block, 1991; Molnar, 1978). The need for normal postural reflex and muscle tone development is also well documented in the disabling condition of cerebral palsy. In cerebral palsied individuals, it is the muscle tone deficits and postural reflexes that inhibit basic postural development and so interfere with acquisition of normal locomotor patterns (Bobath, 1985; Leonard, Hirschfeld and Forssberg, 1991).

In summary, sensory integration and postural stability are important processes. These integrative processes underlie all movement behaviour, and still influence more mature movement behaviour and performance of complex skills, even when children have acquired greater cognitive control over their movements (Trevarthen, 1984). Advanced control of movement will be discussed in the next sections.

Motor learning and control processes (advanced processes)

There are two broad approaches to explaining how we learn and control movements. The first, motor learning theory, stresses the importance of sensory information and central representation of movement. The other, motor control theory, minimizes the role of sensory representation (Abernathy and Sparrow, 1992). Both approaches attempt to explain the manner by which well learnt movements are performed using similar units of movement on different occasions. In addition, they must explain how we are able to produce novel movements that we have never performed before. Each of these major cognitive theories will be discussed.

Overview of motor learning

Motor learning theorists are of the opinion that sensory information is very important to our ability to learn and control movement. This is because it provides the information for central representation of movement in motor memory and in motor schemas. In theory, such a mechanism allows for the enhancement and interpretation of movement received through the senses (Haggard, 1992; Marteniuk, MacKenzie and Leavitt, 1988).

When people are learning any new skill their primary concern is with acquiring the movements necessary to perform it. Practice leads to refinement of the actions and the phasing (timing between the different components in the movement), amount of force and the spatial accuracy of the movements (Newell, 1985). In these early stages of acquiring motor skills attention can only be paid to a small aspect of the task, because of limitations in memory mechanisms. Memory limitations are detrimental to the performance of the whole skill when attentional demand is important (Colley and Beech, 1988). This usually means that in newly learnt skills there is a tendency to reduce the complexity of the movement by reducing the number of different components that comprise the movement, including the degree of flexion or rotation of the joints involved in the action. Well learnt skills, in contrast, can be performed with low attentional demand because it is feasible that some aspects of the task can be performed automatically. The implications of increased automation of movement are that far more complex movements can be performed without requiring all the person's attention.

Some aspects of a motor skill may always need ongoing monitoring, so they will still require attention. In running, for example, once the basic movement has been mastered, the ongoing sequence only requires a moderate amount of attention to scan the environment. A great deal of attention need only be paid when the running surface changes, or the action has to be modified. Motor learning theorists employ the concept of a generalized motor programme to explain the manner in which a movement such as running is stored in motor memory and the action is formulated and performed (Keele, 1981; Newell, 1985; Schmidt, 1982, 1988).

Generalized motor programmes are assumed to contain prestructured commands for many movements, that may be varied by applying specific parameters, such as the overall duration, overall force, muscle selection and spatial location, to effect the desired movement (Schmidt, 1988). Some of these parameters Schmidt considered invariant (i.e. they determine the unchanging features of a movement skill), whereas other parameters were classified as variant, as they are used when a movement skill needs to be altered or modified.

Walking, for example, has both variant and invariant features. In walking there is 50% phasing between the alternate actions of the lower limbs (Clark and Whitall, 1989), which is an invariant feature of this movement skill. By changing the overall duration parameter, the entire action can be speeded up or slowed down yet the 50% overall phasing is maintained between the lower limbs. In handwriting the shape of the letters form the invariant feature of the movement but if the overall force parameter is increased then the size of the letters will be larger. If it is decreased then the size of the letters will be smaller. When the muscle selection parameter is varied, the letters with a similar shape to those written by hand could be produced by muscles in the foot, or the mouth. Another parameter, the spatial parameter is used, for instance, when throwing a ball at a target, for whereas the muscular pattern of the throwing movement may remain the same, the direction of the ball can be changed by differing the angle of the shoulder, wrist and elbow joints (Schmidt, 1988).

The concept of a generalized motor programme helps to explain how novel movements can be produced or how well learnt movements can be modified. Yet, it is also necessary to have a theory to help explain how movements are learned. Once again Schmidt's (1988) motor schema theory provides a useful basis for explanation. According to his theory when a movement generated by a generalized motor programme is performed, four aspects of that movement are temporarily stored in memory. These aspects are (1) body position and environmental features relevant to performance of the task; (2) storage of the parameters that were used to perform the movement; (3) the outcome, stored as knowledge of the results of the movement; and (4) the sensory feel of the movement while it was being performed. Once relationships between this temporary information are formed these are stored in memory as recall and recognition schemas. In recall schemas the relationships between the outcomes of the movement and the parameters used to perform it are stored in memory. In recognition schemas the relationships between the initial conditions and the sensory feel of the movement are stored.

According to Schmidt's motor schema theory 'we learn skills by learning rules about the functioning of our bodies, forming relationships between how our muscles are activated, what they actively do and how these actions feel' (Schmidt, 1988, p. 488). Despite the general applicability of his model, Schmidt (1988) is of the opinion that not all aspects of a movement skill are best explained by generalized motor programmes and motor schemas. This is because performance of a complex movement sequence would require too much space in memory, so some aspects of this type of movement are best explained by motor control theory.

Motor learning in children

It has been suggested that as children mature they become better at processing sensory information, and it is this factor that causes some of the age-related changes in motor development. In addition, the reason children appear slower at performing many movement tasks is that their memory is limited in comparison with that of adults. There is evidence that children's memory systems operate more slowly in the perceptual mechanism, in which sensory information is translated into internal representations of a movement and where children have been shown to have less ability to discriminate between various levels of input of sensory information (Gabbard, 1992; Gallagher and Thomas, 1986; Thomas, 1984).

Evidence also exists that encoding, rehearsal and organization of all motor memory functions is less efficient in children under 7 years, than in 11 year olds who, in turn, are less efficient than adults. It has been shown though, that children can be helped to learn a specific skill more effectively if they are provided with the strategy to assist them to remember the components of the skill (Thomas, 1984). In addition, because information in memory is derived from experience, in order to improve children's movement skills it is very important to provide a wide base of experiences for young children. This implies that it is better to provide general movement experiences for children than only to teach them specific skills.

Deficits in children's memory have important implications for the speed with which children can process movement-related information and for the number of components of a task which they can combine into a smooth sequence. One of the logical consequences of improved information processing ability in older children is that they become better at learning and controlling ongoing movement sequences and so are able to perform and learn more complex sequences of skilled movements.

Motor control processes

Motor control is becoming a distinct area, from motor learning, within the field of research in human movement (Abernathy and Sparrow, 1992). Although theorists in the area of motor control may differ from one another, most are of the opinion that control of movement is a result of the interaction between the person performing the movement and environmental conditions. The majority are also of the opinion that perception and action cannot be be studied separately and that movements are not controlled by memory traces within the central nervous system (e.g. Turvey and Kugler, 1984). This is the major reason why there is little or no emphasis in motor control theory on how sensory information is stored within the central nervous system (Marteniuk, MacKenzie and Leavitt, 1988). Instead, researchers in the field of motor control are seeking a theoretical framework which delineates the 'language of movement' (Stelmach and Diggles, 1982, p. 83).

Bernstein (1967), a prominent early researcher in the area of motor control, was of the opinion that the understanding of motor coordination required knowledge of the constraints, or the ways in which joint combinations are selected from the large repertoire of possible combinations. This reduction of the degrees of freedom for movement of any joint combination was explained by Bernstein in terms of neurological factors resulting in linkages of groups of muscles into units of action. That is to say, the individual achieves control over the many possible muscle actions of the body, by grouping them into an organized system of constraints (Newell, 1985).

Researchers in the area since Bernstein claim that these constraints consist of synergies or muscle linkages which are derived from mechanical constraints of the limb and body segments (Greene, 1982), or from neurally based synergies (Lee, 1984). Some of these synergies are derived from reflexive movements (Easton, 1977). Still other synergies have been identified that maintain postural stability or that control the flexion and extension action of the arm and wrists (Greene, 1982; Hinton, 1984; Nashner, 1976; Nashner, Black and Wall, 1982). Synergies produce a predetermined movement pattern, such as that seen in the early phases of interlimb coordination in walking running jumping, catching and throwing.

According to action theorists, cognitive control of movement is achieved by a neural system with multiple levels of control. The motor cortex represents the level of control where abstract representations of a movement are formulated and where interactions occur among sensory information, integrative and perceptual processes (Arbib, 1984). In addition, Arbib was of the opinion that control is achieved by a number of interacting synergies within the central nervous system to produce the desired movement (Arbib, 1980, 1984). As an example, he cites that even in the simple act of walking down the street with another person there is an interaction of synergies, which helps maintain postural stability, breathing, talking, gesticulating and visual scanning of the environment. In other words he is proposing a holistic notion of motor control (see also, Reed, 1982; Turvey, Shaw and Mace, 1978).

The lower level of control is where abstract movement representations are translated into units of action (to use Bernstein's term). This level of control is often at the spinal cord and is characterized by muscle linkages forming units of action, or synergies which are derived from reflex movements, from muscular and skeletal constraints and from learned movement sequences. The importance of the concept of synergies is that it helps explain how the possible number of movement options, which need to be controlled during a complex movement is reduced, and hence decreases the processing load on the central nervous system. Evidence for the existence of such synergies has been found in locomotor studies (e.g. Patla, 1985; Winter, 1983).

PHASES OF MOTOR CONTROL

The final section of this chapter discusses phases of motor control which are based on an ecological approach to motor learning and control. According to this approach the authors are of the opinion that the movement hierarchy and the sensory-neurological, integrative-perceptual, motor learning-control processes can be conceptualized as three phases of motor control.

In the first phase (sensory-motor phase) children utilize sensory feedback to learn about their environment and to acquire basic control of movement. The second phase (perceptual-motor phase) involves integrative processes resulting in a greater knowledge of the body and a better ability to control it while interacting in the environment. This phase is characterized by an increased ability in processing information from internal and external sources and in planning a motor response (Keogh, 1977). The third phase (cognitive-motor phase) involves learning and advanced control of movement and particularly of the spatial–temporal aspects of complex movements (Keogh and Sugden, 1985).

Sensory-motor phase

The first phase of movement control is demonstrated when young children acquire basic control over the effects of gravity. Such control is demonstrated by developmental milestones such as sitting and crawling. More advanced postural stability and basic movement control are even more crucial for the acquisition of locomotor and manipulative sequences of movement. To achieve these movements children utilize early reflex behaviour, internal and external sensory information and basic movement patterns to learn about their bodies and their environment.

Perceptual-motor phase

Children who are in the perceptual-motor phase of development have sufficient knowledge and experience in movement situations to have developed body awareness including the awareness that the body has two sides (left and right) and the body can be moved in different directions such as up, down, sideways, forwards and backwards. In this phase children also develop spatial awareness in relation to their own bodies and to external objects. Moreover, they have greater visual–spatial awareness, enabling judgements to be made about speed and direction of moving objects and accurate manipulation of tools. Changes in the fundamental movement patterns occur in this second phase because there is greater control of the limbs and postural stability as well as early control of the visual–spatial parameters of movement.

Cognitive-motor phase

Attainment of the third phase of motor development is shown in the acquisition of more complex movement skills, which involves processing relevant external environmental information, as well as controlling the spatial and temporal aspects of the response. These skills are used increasingly by children in their sport and recreational activities. For example, in order to intercept a moving ball children need to process complex visual information while at the same time achieving precise control over the position of their torso and limbs and over the timing of their movement.

In summary, in the first phase of motor control children develop basic awareness of and a rudimentary ability to control their body. In the second phase they increase their level of control of their body and so perform more complex movements in response to external demands. Achievement of advanced control in the third phase, in turn, increases the potential quality and range of movement skills.

CHAPTER SUMMARY

This overview of normal motor development has provided a framework to understand and interpret some of the major changes that occur in the observable hierarchy of movement behaviour as children develop. Some of the underlying behavioural processes that have contributed to these changes have been identified as sensory-neurological, integrative-perceptual, motor learning and control processes. It has been assumed that less mature movements rely on the two earlier processes, whereas advanced control of movement is a synthesis of motor learning and control. An ecological approach is accepted by many authors in the field of motor learning and control. Such a model explains motor learning and motor control in the context of the particular experiences the environment affords (Colley and Beech, 1988; Marteniuk, Mackenzie and Leavitt, 1988; Newell, 1985; Schmidt,1988). The approach adopted incorporates the concept that the units of action or synergies are stored in a generalized motor programme. In young children these early synergies are based on reflexes. With increased maturity well learned and automated units of action, together with postural synergies and biomechanical constraints, are used when performing a sequence of movements. The notion of phases of motor control is discussed in this book is dependent on understanding the framework outlined above. The proposed phases of motor control will be used, particularly in Chapter 7, as a basis for developing guidelines and devising practical activities for children who are clumsy, intellectually disabled or have Down syndrome.

REFERENCES

Abernathy, B. and Sparrow, W.A. (1992) The rise and fall of dominant paradigms in motor behaviour research, *Approaches to the Study of Motor Control and Learning* (ed. J.J. Summers), North Holland, Elsevier, Amsterdam, pp. 3–43.

Abrahams, V.C. (1982) Neck muscle proprioception and motor control, *Proprioception, Posture and Emotion* (ed. D. Garlick), Adept Printing, Bankstown, pp. 103–20.

Ames, L.B. and Ilg, F.L. (1964) The developmental point of view with special reference to the principle of reciprocal neuromotor interweaving. *Journal of Genetic Psychology*, **105**, 95–209.

Ames, L.B. and Ilg, F. (1966) Individuality in motor development. *Journal of the American Physical Therapy Association*, **46**, 121–7.

Arbib, M.A. (1980) Interacting schemas for motor control, in *Tutorials in Motor Behavior* (eds G.E. Stelmach and J.E. Requin), North-Holland, Amsterdam, pp. 71–82.

Arbib, M.A. (1984) From synergies and embryos to motor schemas, in *Human Motor Actions: Bernstein Reassessed* (ed. H.T.A. Whiting), North Holland, Elsevier Science, Amsterdam.

Ayres, A.J. (1982) *Sensory Integration and the Child*, Western Psychological Services, Los Angeles.

Bernstein, N. (1967) *The Coordination and Regulation of Movement*, Pergamon, London.

Block, M. E. (1991) Motor development in children with Down syndrome: a review of literature. *Adapted Physical Activity Quarterly*, **8**, 179–209.

Bobath, K. (1985) *A Neurophysiological Basis for the Treatment of Cerebral Palsy*, William Heinmann, London.

Bruininks, R. (1978) *Bruininks–Oseretsky Test of Motor Proficiency: Examiners Manual*, American Guidance Service, Minnesota.

Burton, A.W. and Davis, W.E. (1992) Assessing balance in adapted physical education: fundamental concepts and applications. *Adapted Physical Activity Quarterly*, **9**, 14–46.

Cameron-Tucker, H. (1983) The neurophysiology of tone: the role of the muscle spindle and stretch reflex. *Australian Journal of Physiotherapy*, **29**(5), 155–65.

Charlton, J.L. (1992) Motor control considerations for assessment and rehabilitation of movement disorders, in *Approaches to the Study of Motor Control and Learning*, (ed. J.J. Summers), North Holland, Elsevier Science, Amsterdam, pp. 3–43.

Clark, J.E., Whitall, J. (1989) Changing patterns of locomotion: from walking to skipping, in *Development of Posture and Gait Across the Life Span*, (ed. M.H. Woollacott and A. Shumway-Cook), University of Southern California, Columbia, pp. 125–51.

Colley, A.M. and Beech, J.R. (1988) Grounds for reconciliation: some preliminary thoughts on cognition and action, in *Cognition and Action in Skilled Behaviour*, (eds A.M. Colley and J.R. Beech), North Holland, Elsevier Science, Amsterdam, pp. 397–403.

Connolly, K. (1980) The development of competence in motor skills, in *Scientific Foundations of Developmental Psychiatry*, (ed. M. Rutter), William Heinemann, London, 138–53.

Daniels, L. and Worthingham, C. (1980) *Muscle Testing: Techniques of Manual Examination*, W.B. Saunders, Philadelphia.

Davis, W.E. and Kelso, J.A.S. (1982) Analysis of 'invariant characteristics' in the motor control of Down's syndrome and normal subjects. *Journal of Motor Behavior*, **14**, 194–212.

Easton, T.A. (1977) Coordinative structures: the basis for a motor program, in *Psychology of Motor Behavior and Sport*, (eds. D.M. Landers and R.W. Christina), Human Kinetics, Champaign, IL, pp. 63–90.

Eliasson, A., Gordon, A.M. and Forssberg, H. (1991) Basic coordination of manipulative forces of children with cerebral palsy. *Develpmental Medicine and Child Neurology*, **33**, 661–70.

Fiorentino, M.R. (1974) *Reflex Testing Methods for Evaluating CNS Development*. Thomas, Springfield, IL.

Fischer, K.W. and Farrar, M .J. (1988) Generalizations about generalizations: how a theory of skill development explains both generality and specificity, in *The Neo-Piagetian Theories of Cognitive Development: Towards an Integration*, (ed A. Demetriou), North-Holland, Elsevier, Amsterdam, pp. 137–71.

Gabbard, C. (1992) *Lifelong Motor Development*, Wm. C. Brown, Dubuque, IA.

Gallagher, J.D. and Thomas, J.R. (1986) Developmental effects of grouping and recoding on learning a movement series. *Research Quarterly for Exercise and Sport*, **57**, 117–27.

Gesell, A.(1978) *The First Five Years of Life*, Methuen, London.

Glencross, D.J. (1980) Levels and strategies of response organization, in *Tutorials in Motor Behavior*, (eds G.E. Stelmach and J. Requin), North Holland, Amsterdam, 551–556.

Greene, P.H. (1982) Why is it easy to control your arms? *Journal of Motor Behavior*, **14**, 260–86.

Haggard, P. (1992) Multisensory control of coordinated movement, in *Approaches to the Study of Motor Control and Learning*, (ed

J.J. Summers), Elsevier Science, Amsterdam, pp. 195–231.
Hinton, G. (1984) Parallel computations for controlling an arm. *Journal of Motor Behavior*, **16**, 171–94.
Holt, K.S. (1975) *Movement and Child Development*, William Heinemann, London.
Horak, F.B., Shumway-Cook, A., Crowe, T.K. and Black, F.O. (1988) Vestibular function and motor proficiency of children with impaired hearing or with learning disability and motor impairments. *Developmental Medicine and Child Neurology*, **30**, 64–79.
Jones, B. (1981) The development of intermodal co-ordination and motor control, in *The Development of Movement Control and Co-ordination*, (ed. J.E. Clark), Wiley, Chichester, pp. 95–109.
Keele, S.W. (1981) Behavioural analysis of movement, in *Handbook of Physiology*. Section 1: The Nervous System, Vol II, Motor Control, Part 2, (ed. V.B. Brooks), American Physiological Society, Baltimore, pp. 1391–414.
Keogh, J.F. (1977) The study of movement skill development. *Quest*, Monograph **28**, 76–86.
Keogh, J. and Sugden, D. (1985) *Movement Skill Development*, Macmillan, New York.
Lazlo, J.I. and Bairstow, P.J. (1982) Tests of kinesthetic sensitivity: kinesthesis in normal development and physical disability, in *Proprioception, Posture and Emotion*, (ed. D. Garlick), Adept Printing, Bankstown, pp. 214–23.
Lazlo, J.I. and Bairstow, P.J. (1985) *Perceptual-Motor Behaviour: Developmental Assessment and Therapy*, Holt, Rinehart and Winston, London.
Lee, W.A. (1984) Neuromotor synergies as a basis for coordinated intentional action. *Journal of Motor Behavior*, **16**, 135–70.
Leonard, C.T., Hirschfeld, H. and Forssberg, H. (1991) The development of independent walking in children with cerebral palsy. *Developmental Medicine and Child Neurology*, **33**, 557–67.
Levitt, S. (1979) *Treatment of Cerebral Palsy and Motor Delay*, J.B. Lippincott, Philadelphia.
Lydic, J.S. and Steele, C. (1979) Assessment of the quality of sitting and gait patterns in children with Down's syndrome. *Physical Therapy*, **59**, 1489–94.
Malina, R.M. (1984) Physical growth and maturation, in *Development During Childhood and Adolescence*, (ed. J.R. Thomas), Burgess, Minneapolis, pp. 2–26.
Martenuink, R.G., Mackenzie, D.L. and Leavitt, J.L. (1988) Representational and physical accounts of motor control and learning: can they account for the data? in *Cognition and Action in Skilled Behaviour*, (eds. A.M. Colley and J.R. Beech), North Holland, Elsevier Science, Amsterdam, pp. 173–90.
McGraw, M.B. (1966) *The Neuromuscular Maturation of the Human*

Infant, Hafner, New York.
Molnar, G.D. (1978) Analysis of motor disorder in retarded infants and young children. *American Journal of Mental Deficiency*, **83**, 213–22.
Nashner, L.M. (1976) Adapting reflexes controlling the human posture. *Experimental Brain Research*, **26**, 59–72.
Nashner, L.M., Black, O. and Wall, C. (1982) Adaptation to altered support and visual conditions during stance: patients with vestibular deficits. *Journal of Neurosciences*, **2**, 536–52.
Newell, K.M. (1984) Physical constraints to development of motor skills, in *Motor Development During Childhood and Adolescence*, (ed. J.R. Thomas), Burgess, Minneapolis, pp. 105–20.
Newell, K.M. (1985) Coordination, control and skill, in *Differing Perspectives in Motor Learning, Memory and Control*, (eds D. Goodman, R.B. Willberg and L.M. Franks), North Holland, Elsevier Science, Amsterdam, pp. 295–317.
O'Brien, C.C. (1991) *Motor Development in Young Children*, V.R. Ward, Government Printer, Brisbane.
O'Brien, C.C. (1994) Motor development and learning in children, in *The Early Years*, (eds. G. Boulton-Lewis and D. Catherwood), The Australian Council for Educational Research, Victoria, Australia, pp. 145–85.
O'Brien, C.C. and Ziviani, J. (1991) *Fine Motor Development and Young Children*, V.R. Ward, Government Printer, Brisbane.
O'Brien, C.C., Parker, A.W., Kennedy, J.M. *et al.* (1993) The development of strategies for the integration of all children in school physical education and sport. Paper presented at *The 9th International Symposium on Adapted Physical Activity*, Yokohama, Japan, August, 1993.
Patla, A.E. (1985) Some characteristics of E.M.G. patterns during locomotion: implications for the locomotor control process. *Journal of Motor Behavior*, **17**, 443–61.
Prechtl, H.F. (1986) Prenatal motor development, in *Motor Development in Children: Aspects of Coordination and Control* (eds M.G. Wade and H.T.A. Whiting), Martinus Nijhoff, Dordretch, pp. 53–64.
Reed, E.S. (1982) An outline of a theory of action systems. *Journal of Motor Behavior*, **14**, 93–134.
Roberton, M.A. (1984) Changing motor patterns during childhood, in *Motor Development During Childhood and Adolescence* (ed. J.R. Thomas, Burgess, Minneapolis, pp. 48–90.
Rochat, P. (1992) Self-sitting and reaching in 5- to 8-month old infants: the impact of posture and its development on early eye–hand coordination. *Journal of Motor Behavior*, **24**, 210–20.
Schmidt, R.A. (1982) *Motor Control and Learning*, Human Kinetics, Champaign, IL.
Schmidt, R.A. (1988) *Motor Control and Learning*, 2nd edn. Human Kinetics, Champaign, IL.
Shepherd, R.B. (1980) Problem analysis with Down's syndrome

infants. *Cumberland College Reports*, Sydney, **20**, 1–14.
Shirley, M.M. (1931) *The First Two Years*. University of Minnesota Press, Minneapolis.
Stelmach, E. and Diggles, V.A. (1982) Control theories in motor behavior. *Acta Psychologica*, **50**, 83–105.
Thelen, E. (1983) Learning to walk is still an 'old' problem: a reply to Zelazo (1983). *Journal of Motor Behavior*, **15**, 139–61.
Thomas, J.R. (1984) Children's motor skill development, in *Motor Development During Childhood and Adolescence*, (ed. J.R. Thomas), Burgess, Minneapolis, pp. 91–104.
Touwen, B. (1976) *Neurological Development in Infancy*. William Heinemann, London.
Trevarthen, C. (1984) How control of movement develops, in *Human Motor Actions: Bernstein Reassessed*, (ed. H.T.A. Whiting), North Holland, Elsevier Science, Amsterdam, pp. 223–61.
Turvey, M.T. and Kugler, P.N. (1984) An ecological approach to perception and action, in *Tutorials in Motor Behavior* (eds G.E. Stelmach and J.E. Requin), North-Holland, Amsterdam, pp. 373–412.
Turvey, M.T., Shaw, R.E. and Mace, W. (1978) Issues in the theory of action, degrees of freedom, coordinative structures and coalitions. *Attention and Performance*, **7**, 557–95.
van Wierington, P.C.C. (1986) Motor coordination: constraints and cognition, in *Motor Development in Children: Aspects of Coordination and Control* (eds M.G. Wade and H.T.A. Whiting), Martinus Nijhoff, Dordrecht, pp. 361–9.
Walsh, G. (1992) *Muscles, Masses and Motion: The Physiology of Normality, Spasticity and Rigidity*. Blackwell Scientific Publications, Oxford.
White, B.L. (1970) Experience and the development of motor mechanisms in infancy, in *Mechanisms of Motor Skill Development*, (ed. K.J. Connolly), Academic Press, London, pp. 95–133.
Winter, D.A. (1983) Biomechanical motor patterns in normal walking. *Journal of Motor Behavior*, **15**, 302–30.
Wolf, P.H. (1986) The maturation and development of fetal motor patterns, in *Motor Development in Children: Aspects of Coordination and Control* (eds M.G. Wade and H.T.A. Whiting), Martinus Nijhoff, Dordrecht, pp. 65–74.
Woollacott, M.H., Shumway-Cook, A. and Williams, H.G. (1989) The development of posture and balance control in children, in *Development of Posture and Gait Across the Life Span* (eds M.H. Woollacott and A. Shumway-Cook), University of Southern California, Columbia, pp. 77–96.
Wyke, B. (1976) Neurological mechanisms in spasticity. A brief review of some current concepts. *Physical Therapy*, **62**, 316–19.
Yokochi, K., Shimabukuro, S., Kodama, M. *et al.* (1993) Motor

functions of infants with athetoid cerebral palsy. *Developmental Medicine and Child Neurology*, **35**, 909–16.
Zelazo, P.R. (1983) The development of walking: new findings on old assumptions. *Journal of Motor Behavior*, **2**, 99–137.
Zernicke, R.F., Gregor, R.J. and Cratty, B.J. (1982) Balance and visual proprioception in children. *Journal of Human Movement Studies*, **8**, 1–13.

2

Motor development in movement impaired children

In this chapter motor impairment will be explored by examining the behaviour of children who are clumsy, or intellectually disabled or have Down syndrome. The aim is to determine what delay or difference there is in the movement behaviour of these children by focusing on their sensory-neurological, perceptual-motor and cognitive-motor development. The final section discusses why it is important to use multiple measures of movement behaviour and outlines suitable assessment instruments that may be used by practitioners.

THE ISSUE OF DEVELOPMENTAL DELAY VERSUS DIFFERENCE

Although the normal development of children has been shown to follow a relatively predictable pattern (Boulton-Lewis and Catherwood, 1994; Fischer and Farrer, 1988; Fischer and Lazerson, 1984; Fischer and Silvern, 1985), it is uncertain whether children who have not acquired normal skills for their age progress through the sequences in the same manner (Hayes, 1990).

There are two opposing assumptions about development in children who have not acquired normal skills. The first assumption is that their development is delayed and they will progress through developmental sequences in a similar fashion, but at a slower rate. This is known as the developmental delay position. It implies that the biological factors which control the progression of the immature organism to a mature state are delayed, and so slow down the rate of development (Anastasiow, 1986). The second assumption is that children with cognitive or motor handicaps have some deficit which will cause them to show differences in the pattern of their development (Touwen, 1990; Zigler and Hodapp, 1986). This is referred to as the developmental difference position. It implies that there are differences in the biological processes of some children that will change both the speed and the manner of their development.

The problem of delay versus difference in development has important applied ramifications. Specifically, it has implications both for developmental assessment and for intervention. For instance, delay implies that development progresses at a slower rate but follows a pattern similar to that of normally developing children. If delay is demonstrated then children should be provided with enrichment programmes, at their own developmental level, to encourage progression to the next level. Conversely, developmental difference implies that although the children concerned may achieve many of the developmental milestones and skills of normally developing children, they achieve them in a different manner, or in a different sequence from their normally developing peers. For example, children with Down syndrome may achieve the developmental milestone of sitting by adopting a posture with their legs very wide apart. This posture inhibits progression to other milestones that require the child to rotate sideways to achieve a crawling position on the hands and knees, which in turn leads to pulling, to standing and then to upright walking. In other words attaining a developmental milestone in this manner will actually inhibit normal progression to more advanced levels of movement.

Children who are developing differently, therefore, may require specific intervention techniques in order to achieve important developmental sequences and skills. Some children may be both developmentally delayed and different. These children will need an intervention programme which includes activities specially devised to address delayed aspects of their development, but at the same time ensuring that their particular areas of developmental difference are also addressed.

When trying to assess children with disabilities the concept of developmental delay is a simpler one than that of developmental difference. This is because if the developmental delay hypothesis is accepted as the explanation of a problem in such children, then all that needs to be determined is the extent of the delay. Once the extent of the delay is determined it is possible to implement programmes suitable for the child's current level of development, based on knowledge of patterns of development and children, generally. In contrast, the developmental difference hypothesis requires more specific evaluation techniques in order to determine the nature and extent of differences and the optimum techniques to use in intervention programmes.

The design of appropriate intervention depends on the availability of two types of information. The first is about a child's specific problems derived from individual assessment. The second type of information is derived from relevant literature and current research about the types of problems these children are likely to experience. Because assessment of motor impaired children requires a multiple measure approach, the next section in this chapter will discuss the motor behaviour measures used in a series of studies by the authors. The studies were designed to validate assessment protocols and to ascertain specific motor problems found in children who are clumsy intellectually disabled or have Down syndrome. Another reason for the studies was to determine if each of the groups of children have similar as well as specific problems associated with their motor impairment. A subsequent section will review relevant literature to determine general problems which have been identified in these disabled children.

INFORMATION DERIVED FROM ASSESSMENT INSTRUMENTS

Whether children's development is seen as delayed or different may depend on the instrument used to assess their behaviour (Hallam *et al.*, 1993; Maeland, 1992). Age-referenced tests of performance, for example, may give the impression of delay because they can only be interpreted in terms of a child's position relative to the mean level of performance for a particular age. Since specific tests give a different impression of the child's problems, it is important to examine different facets of development if a more holistic picture is to be obtained. It is possible for instance to take multiple measures of the aspect of development being studied to gain a more balanced, comprehensive assessment of each child's development. For these reasons each test that was used in the studies and the advantages and disadvantages of each of the measures will be discussed.

Motor performance

The first aspect, motor performance, was chosen to measure motor behaviour. The authors decided to determine the children's levels of motor performance by using the Bruininks-Oseretsky Test of Motor Proficiency (Bruininks, 1978). This test was chosen because they had used it successfully for many years to gain information about the relative standing of children who are clumsy, intellectually disabled or who have Down syndrome, when compared against age norms (for more details on why this instrument was chosen, see Appendix A).

Motor performance tests provide quantitative measures of motor behaviour, such as how far children can run, jump or throw, how many successful catches they make or how long they can balance in a certain posture. The performance is scored in terms of predetermined speed, time, or distance criteria (Rarick, 1981, 1982). The major advantage of motor performance tests is that they provide quantitative, normative data on children which enables the assessor to decide whether a particular child's motor performance is average, or above or below age norms. A disadvantage of this type of test is that it is norm-referenced (usually by age) so this type of the assessment may maximize the impression of delay. As argued above, each child's scores can only be interpreted in terms of their relative standing when compared with the norms for children of similar chronological age (Davis, 1984; Henderson, 1987).

The tasks that motor performance tests measure are also very dependent on whether children can understand the task, or are sufficiently motivated to produce their best performance. For example, the Bruininks–Oseretsky Test of Motor Proficiency, which children, and particularly those who are intellectually disabled, have to be taught to perform, requires them to place the heel of their forward foot against the toes on their back foot while maintaining balance on the beam. A related problem is that the assessment does not provide information about whether a failure to perform the task is due to lack of motivation or deficits in underlying motor processes. Furthermore, motor performance tests do not provide information about the maturity of children's fundamental movement patterns while performing the set task. The authors considered it was necessary, therefore, to develop an assessment instrument which examined the maturity of the children's fundamental movement patterns.

Fundamental movement patterns

Fundamental movement patterns were the second aspect of movement behaviour to be studied. The pattern of fundamental movements is regarded as a measure of motor development which is suitable for criterion-referenced assessment. Criterion-referenced assessment is a useful diagnostic tool because it provides information about the child's competencies and deficiencies and so can be related more directly to activities which should be included in an adapted motor programme for that particular child (Reid, 1985). It is also regarded as less obtrusive because the predetermined levels of movement behaviour enable the observer to study children in naturalistic situations, with no requirements for them to perform specific skills under the assessor's direction.

As a measure, the Fundamental Movement Pattern Checklist (developed by O'Brien, 1988; for details see Chapter 5) is sensitive to experiential influences, since it has been shown that mature levels of the movement patterns are not attained if children do not practise them (Halverson, Roberton and Langendorfer, 1982; Wickstrom, 1983). In addition, it is a qualitative measure of movement which allows observation of the manner in which children maintain their postural stability, coordinate their limbs and control their movements (Thelen, 1986).

Some disadvantages associated with the measurement of fundamental movement patterns are that they are subjective measures and, as such, are dependent upon the knowledge and observational skills of the person using them. In addition, the assessor needs considerable training or experience to be able to use them in a naturalistic situation without having to refer to lengthy descriptions.

Motor control

One of the issues in the motor learning and control literature that is applicable to increased movement skill levels and motor patterns, is how children control their limb movements. This was the third aspect of movement behaviour to be examined by the authors. Techniques such as the interlimb coordination task, as reported in this book, attempt to measure underlying motor learning-control processes which affect movement behaviour. Such studies generally have been neglected in children, yet they are very important. They provide information about interlimb constraints, the timing and accuracy of movements and the speed of making a motor response (Newell and Barclay, 1982; Zelaznick, 1986).

Motor control studies in children should seek to measure processes which enable better coordination and hence better quality of movement. If there is a problem, for example, in timing or force control, then the child will probably have jerky and inappropriate movements. A major disadvantage with measures of motor control, like motor performance tests, is that children must have the cognitive ability to understand the task, and in addition, must be motivated to perform the task to the best of their ability (Smyth, 1986).

In conclusion, the above discussion of advantages and disadvantages of the three measures of motor behaviour emphasizes the value of assessing more than one aspect of movement behaviour. Similarly, it is contended that multiple measures, such as the ones that have been discussed, are needed to develop appropriate adapted physical activity programmes for motor impaired children (e.g. Davis, 1984; Hardin and Garcia, 1982; O'Brien, 1988; Maeland, 1992).

The results from the studies using the above three measures, separately, to examine motor performance, fundamental movement patterns and motor control, are reported in Chapters 3, 5 and 6, respectively.

MOTOR DEVELOPMENT AND CHARACTERISTICS OF CLUMSY CHILDREN

Clumsy children defined

A currently accepted definition of clumsiness is that these children cannot perform culturally normative motor skills, even though there are no abnormal signs on routine neurological examination. There is also no diagnosis of ataxia, involuntary movement, weakness, sensory loss or spasticity (Gubbay, 1989, p.14). Despite the absence of severe neurological deficits, the extent of their coordination problems are such that they have difficulties performing many everyday skills (van der Meulen *et al.*, 1991).

Clumsiness has often been used as a relative term, based on normal movement behaviour. For example, toddlers learning to walk, run and jump exhibit clumsy movement behaviour in their jerky, hesitant movements and frequent falls. This type of behaviour is accepted as normal for toddlers but the same type of movement behaviour three years later (in preschool children) is regarded as clumsy.

There are many reasons for clumsiness. It may be an early indication of more serious medical problems and the condition will get worse (progressive), or it may be a symptom of a problem that will not become worse (non-progressive) (Gubbay, 1975; Henderson, 1987). Examples of progressive deficits in children include brain tumours, poisoning by external agents such as lead, mercury and DDT, drug toxicity, muscular dystrophy and muscular atrophy. Non-progressive defects which may cause clumsiness in children include cerebral palsy; visual problems such as squint, astigmatism or uncorrected faulty vision; orthopaedic problems; intellectual handicap; minimal brain damage; and developmental apraxia (Gordon and McKinlay, 1980; Gubbay, 1975, 1989). Although non-progressive clumsiness does not appear to worsen these children appear to have persistent problems in their school years (Losse *et al.*, 1991).

Recently it has been shown that children identified with neurodevelopmental disorders at 6–7 years of age still have minor motor control problems and delay in complex visual reactions ten years later even though the outcome for some of the children was within the normal range (Hellegren *et al.*, 1993). Another study has shown that 50% of children who were aged between 6 and 11 years, in a study five years earlier, still had persistent fine and gross motor problems, even though they were then aged 11–17 years (Geuze and Borger, 1993). The results from both these studies would suggest that many children, identified with neurodevelopmental deficits, retain motor control problems in adolescence, despite popular belief that they will grow out of their problems.

The primary concern in this book is the movement behaviour of two specific types of clumsy children. Children who are often recognized by the medical profession as having a syndrome called developmental apraxia, or the clumsy child syndrome and other children who have coordination problems but no 'soft neurological signs' (Gubbay, 1975, 1978, 1989; Smyth, 1992). Children with the clumsy child syndrome may be of average or near average intelligence, but they have minor neurological problems such as associated movements consisting of small, jerky, irregular movements of the fingers and wrist, delayed laterality and borderline electroencephalogram abnormalities, as well as impaired timing of movements and abnormal postural reactions (Geuze and Kalverboer, 1987; Gubbay, 1975, 1978; Lazarus and Todor, 1991; Williams, Woollacott and Ivry, 1992).

The other group of children who do not appear to have overt neurological problems are still classified by neurologists as clumsy on a subjective examination. In this type of examination children are usually required to perform tasks such as hopping, doing jigsaw puzzles, tying shoe laces and writing. These clumsy children, who may only have a coordination problem, are likely to experience failure and frustration in the playground. Their motor problems may also seriously affect their ability to speak and, if they have a fine motor problem as well, they will have difficulty with all forms of manual skills, so the motor problem is often only one of many problems which may be present in clumsy children (Bullock and Watter, 1987; Gillberg, 1985; Gordon and McKinlay, 1980; Larkin and Hoare, 1991).

In terms of motor performance these children have been shown to have difficulty with static and dynamic balance, ball skills, manual dexterity, gross motor control, fine motor control and production of simultaneous movements (Henderson and Hall, 1982; O'Brien and Hayes, 1989; Parker and Bronks, 1986). Many also have specific learning disabilities related to reading, spelling and arithmetic, and they are likely to have problems with behaviour, speech and writing (Gordon and McKinlay, 1980; Gillberg, 1985; Gillberg, Gillberg and Groth, 1989; Henderson *et al.*, 1991; Smyth, 1992).

The prognosis for many of these children is that they may have difficulties well into adolescence. Of those children diagnosed with motor perceptual dysfunction and/or attentional deficit disorder at age 7 years, 25% will have major learning problems and behaviour problems at 10 years (Gillberg, 1985). The learning problem will increase to the extent that about 40% will have learning problems at 13 years, whereas only 17% will exhibit behaviour problems. Finally, it has been claimed that any 13-year old who has motor clumsiness will most probably have motor perception dysfunction and may also have attentional deficit disorder or some other neurological dysfunction (Gillberg, Gillberg and Groth, 1989). The majority of these children do not have major neurological abnormalities, but their clumsiness may still be so severe that it interferes with daily living skills, more so than in many children who are diagnosed as having mild cerebral palsy.

Motor development in clumsy children

In the non-progressive clumsy syndrome it is clear that many of the children suffer from apparent neurological dysfunction which manifests itself behaviourally in coordination problems, learning disabilities and neurologically 'soft signs' such as jerky, irregular movements, squint, delayed laterality, sensory dysfunction, poorly timed movements, and learning disabilities. There is another group of children who have non-specific clumsiness, but still find it difficult to plan or execute movements. They may also have a generalized lack of strength (Gubbay, 1975, 1989; Larkin and Hoare, 1992; Marchiori, Wall and Bedingfield, 1987).

The effect of these problems on clumsy children has mainly been studied by using therapeutic and medical paradigms. Bullock and Watter (1987), for instance, reported that young children with minimal cerebral dysfunction, who exhibited movement problems as babies, still had movement problems as toddlers and in early childhood. There have also been some comprehensive Scandinavian Studies (Gillberg, 1985; Gillberg, Gillberg and Groth, 1989; Rasmussen *et al.*, 1983) which have shown that children who were diagnosed as having minimal brain dysfunction had coordination problems until they were about 10 years of age. After 10 years of age, physical differences remained between these children and their normal peers and many of them retained learning disorders and behavioural problems (Gillberg, Gillberg and Groth, 1989). Similar problems were still evident five years later (Hellegren *et al.*, 1993).

Apart from Gubbay's (1975, 1978, 1989) work on neurological and medical aspects of clumsiness there is some specific work available on aspects of sensory-neurological, integrative-perceptual, and motor learning-control deficits that will affect movement in clumsy children. There is early evidence, for example, that clumsy children have underlying sensory-neurological deficits that often manifest in delayed developmental milestones. Furthermore, those clumsy children, found to have movement problems as babies, continued to have problems throughout early childhood (Bullock and Watter, 1987).

In terms of integrative-perceptual processes, an extensive study is reported by Hoare and Larkin (1991). They measured kinaesthetic sensitivity, cross-modal matching with vision and kinaesthesis and kinaesthetic perception and memory, in 80 children aged between 6 and 9 years. These children were chosen because they were more than one standard deviation below their age norm on the McCarron Assessment of Neuromuscular Development. The results on perceptual-motor functioning tasks showed that in terms of utilizing movement-related sensory information, 22% of clumsy children were below their normal peers in kinaesthetic perception, 12% had mainly visual problems and 10% had problems across visual and kinaesthetic tasks. These results would suggest that just over half the population of clumsy children is likely to have perceptual problems due to specific sensory areas. Yet only 22% have major problems in the kinaesthetic modality, even though it has often been proposed that children are clumsy because of kinaesthetic modality dysfunction and that kinaesthetic training will improve their coordination (Lazlo and Bairstow, 1985: Lazlo, Bartrip and Rolfe, 1988).

Another study investigated the manner in which clumsy children integrate sensory information (Hulme *et al.*, 1982). It was found that when clumsy children, as identified by Gubbay's (1975, 1978) test, were asked to make cross-modal visual and kinaesthetic judgements about the length of a line, they had great difficulty in translating information from the visual condition. On the basis of this evidence, these authors suggested that poor motor coordination in these children may be partly due to their problems with information processing in regard to distance and spatial relationships. It has also been shown that they have less efficient use of visual feedback in visual tracking tasks than their peers (van der Meulen *et al.*, 1991).

Although the previous research confirms that clumsy children have problems in controlling visual tracking, their dysfunction has been shown to be greater in the kinaesthetic modality when measuring their response in a complex reaction time task. In this type of information-processing task there was no significant difference among all groups of children, who performed the same when they used the visual modality (Smyth, 1991). In addition to possible information processing difficulties, there is some evidence from complex reaction time experiments that clumsy children are slower at programming movement responses. These children may also be more dependent on sensory feedback (Smyth, 1991). These findings imply that clumsy children may also have motor learning and control deficits, especially as other researchers have found them to have slower complex reaction times than their normal peers and the timing and force control of their movements has been shown to be less consistent and adaptable (Geuze and Kalverboer, 1987; Marchiori, Wall and Bedingfield, 1987; O'Brien, 1988, Van Dellen and Geuze, 1988).

This brief literature review has indicated that clumsiness is a general term and children so afflicted have many other symptoms, as well as the observed clumsiness. From the studies reported it is evident that these children may have specific deficits or a combination of deficits in the processes which contribute to their observable movement incoordination.

It is considered important, therefore, to examine multimodal differences in motor development in these children as well as comparing their development with normally developing children, and other groups of motor impaired children.

MOTOR DEVELOPMENT AND CHARACTERISTICS OF INTELLECTUALLY DISABLED CHILDREN

Intellectually disabled children defined

Intellectually disabled children are usually categorized on the basis of the number of standard deviations they are below normal children, in their IQ scores, on intelligence tests (Kirk and Gallagher, 1986; Zigler and Hodapp, 1986). Chromosomal abnormalities, for example, resulting in individuals who have Down syndrome (discussed fully in the next section), are the cause for over a quarter of all intellectual disability. Familial reasons account for the majority of the remaining cases (Sherrill, 1986), whereas factors such as birth trauma, prematurity, infection, metabolic and nutritional disorders are also well-known causes (Kirk and Gallagher, 1986). Intellectually disabled children comprise 3% of the normal population.

As discussed in Chapter 1 there is a debate about whether intellectually disabled children, who do not show signs of organic problems, are merely delayed in their development or whether these children exhibit differences in their development (Touwen, 1990; Zigler and Hodapp, 1986). However, there is consensus that children who have organic or genetic impairment usually develop differently from intellectually disabled children who are classified as familial, or ideopathic. All groups of intellectually disabled children, however, are generally delayed in the rate of their development, in comparison with normal peers.

Motor development in intellectually disabled children

Intellectually disabled children have been found to have deficits in sensory-neurological, integrative-perceptual and motor control processes affecting motor development. In terms of sensory-neurological processes, Molnar (1978) tested intellectually disabled children (ranging in age from 10 to 25 months at the beginning of her study) for reflex behaviour and muscle tone. She found that even though these children did not have abnormalities in tone and postural reflexes, their postural reflexes were delayed when compared with normal infants. Also of interest from her data was the finding that the emergence of primitive reflexes is inhibited in these children. When the delayed postural reflexes appeared they achieved a more mature level of movement behaviour.

Another study that examined basic processing deficits, compared the sensory-motor capacities of normal and intellectually disabled children (Chenoweth and Bullock, 1978). This study found evidence of muscle tone abnormalities and poor body awareness in the intellectually disabled children (of chronological age 10 years and mental age approximately 5 years). The authors also found that these children had sensory-motor abilities similar to those of children of the same mental age. In addition, they were of the opinion that muscle tone abnormalities contributed to their problems of poor dynamic and static balance, as well as to their poor fine and gross motor coordination.

Research into integrative-perceptual processes was conducted on intellectually disabled children (in the mild to moderate range), chronologically aged 13 years, who were matched with normal children with a similar mental age of 8 years (Davidson *et al.*, 1980). These authors found that, in general, intellectually disabled children were able to match shapes, as proficiently as normally developing children of similar mental age. Such a finding is in agreement with the previous study and confirms that in terms of utilizing information these children operate at their mental rather than their chronological age.

Motor learning-control processes have been examined in intellectually disabled individuals (Davis, Sparrow and Ward, 1991; Hoover and Wade, 1985), and it is argued that there has been a great deal of information processing research which suggests that intellectually disabled individuals have slower reaction times than their normal peers. Many of the reviewed studies appear to have assumed that documenting the deficit between the reaction times in persons with intellectual disabilities, and those of non-intellectually disabled individuals, would help explain the characteristic slowness of movement in intellectually disabled children.

Despite this popular belief about the effects on motor skills of the slow reaction time in intellectually disabled invididuals, Hoover and Wade (1985) cite evidence which shows that it is only in relatively unskilled tasks that reaction times may predict performance outcomes. This would mean that information processing capacity limitations may not be the only explanation of the slow and awkward performance of intellectually disabled individuals, on more complex movement tasks. In fact Hoover and Wade (1985) do not believe that reaction time deficits explain the observed coordination problems in intellectually disabled individuals any better than earlier descriptive approaches. Indeed this position that reaction time deficit is not the major cause for motor coordination, is supported by some researchers who are of the opinion that intellectually disabled children have memory and retrieval deficits. They also appear to have an apparent inability to develop cognitive strategies for remembering movement information (Bouffard, 1990; Thomas, 1984).

There is definite evidence that motor development in intellectually disabled children seems delayed when compared with normal children (see Chapter 3, for a review), but it is not clear to what extent this is due to sensory-neurological, integrative-perceptual and motor learning-control processes. Furthermore, apart from observational data of slow movements in these children, it is not known how intellectually disabled children control their movements, or whether they control them in a different way to normal children.

MOTOR DEVELOPMENT AND CHARACTERISTICS OF CHILDREN WITH DOWN SYNDROME

Children with Down syndrome defined

Children with Down syndrome have a chromosomal disorder which has far-reaching effects on their cognitive and physical development. Karyotyping of chromosomes in most persons with Down syndrome shows an extra chromosome number 21, indicating the condition referred to as trisomy 21. Down syndrome is the largest single chromosomally determined intellectually handicapping condition. Children with Down syndrome comprise approximately one third of the intellectually disabled population. There is some evidence of a trend for the intellectual disability of these children, as measured on intelligence tests, to show a steady decline during infancy and childhood. This trend towards a decrease in measures on intelligence tests continues as the child matures, but appears to stabilize at about 11 years of age (Carr, 1992). It should be noted, though, that there are wide individual differences, and previous research showing the decline has been criticized methodologically (Berry, Gunn and Andrews, 1984; Carr, 1992; Hayes and Gunn, 1991).

A decline in the motor development of young children with Down syndrome has also been well documented (e.g. Carr, 1992; Share and French, 1982). In early infancy the motor development of these children is close to normal, but by one year of age they are delayed and this trend continues with increased age. A similar decline in motor performance in children with Down syndrome from about 10 years of age has also been reported by Henderson (1985). Another study found that infants and young children, (aged from birth to 6 years 11 months) who were tested on the Baley Scale of Infant Development showed differences in development from normally developing peers. The children studied passed test items of grasping and reaching earlier than was expected but were later than expected in standing and maintaining postural stability and unaided locomotion (Dyer *et al.*, 1990).

The summary of the literature in the next section will concentrate on the motor development of children with Down syndrome.

Motor development in children with Down syndrome

Children with Down syndrome are often delayed or abnormal in their physical and gross and fine motor development (Block, 1991; Thombs and Sugden, 1991). It has been reported, for example, that nearly half the children with Down syndrome have cardiac abnormalities which are detrimental to their growth and fitness, about 20% have atlantoaxial instability and about 2% of these have marked subluxation of the joint resulting in muscle weakness and increasing loss of motor coordination (Block, 1991). Nearly all children with Down syndrome have joint laxity, hypertonia, myopia (near sightedness), many have problems of impaired visual and auditory acuity and perception (Block, 1991).

From infancy these children demonstrate deficiencies in most areas associated with sensory-neurological processes of motor development, including extension against gravity, orientation and balance of the body, weight shifting and weight bearing (Shepherd, 1980). They also have a longer period in which primitive reflexes dominate their early movement behaviour (Haley, 1986). For example, about a quarter of these children have persistent plantar and palmar reflexes up to 9 months of age. Hyperflexibility and generalized hypotonia (low muscle tone) are evident at birth although they both become less severe as the child grows older (Parker and James, 1985). The presence of hypotonia, together with a later than normal appearance of postural reflexes, delays in postural milestones and locomotor skills is common in these children (Haley, 1986; Harris, 1986; Rast and Harris, 1985; Shepherd, 1980). More recently it has been claimed that as well as having hypotonia, children with Down syndrome have weaknesses in the flexor and extensor muscles which will affect their ability to maintain static and dynamic posture (Shumway-Cook and Woollacott, 1988; Woollacott, 1993).

The persistence of delays and apparent differences in motor development in children with Down syndrome has been attributed to immaturity of the nervous system and decreased growth of the cerebellum and brainstem, which average only 66% of normal growth (Crome, Cowie and Slater, 1966; McIntire and Dutch, 1964). The decreased size of the cerebellum and brainstem is thought to be the major cause of hypotonia at birth. It is also implicated in the persistence of the primitive reflexes and delay in postural reactions, and in addition, it may explain the reported difficulty that these children have in timing their movements. It may also partially explain why infants with Down syndrome have difficulty in maintaining postural tone and muscle tone (Davis and Sinning, 1987).

Perhaps of equal importance is the research relevant to understanding integrative-perceptual processes which has shown that children with Down syndrome have deficits in processing movement-related information. Butterworth and Cicchetti (1978), for example, are of the opinion that these infants experience a feedback discrepancy between the visual and the proprioceptive mechanisms underlying postural stability. Furthermore, they have suggested that an apparent deficit in visual perception may be another contributing factor to their delayed locomotion.

Lazlo and Bairstow (1985) and Bairstow and Lazlo, (1981) have demonstrated that although kinaesthetic awareness is the same as in normal children (i.e. initial sensory reception), children with Down syndrome still have problems with kinaesthetic memory which could indicate a deficit in integrating sensory information. Further evidence of deficits in integrating sensory information has been provided by research into the neuropsychological correlates of information processing in children with Down syndrome (Lincoln *et al.*, 1985). These researchers report evidence which shows that children with Down syndrome may not process auditory information, as efficiently as normally developing children of the same chronological age and the same mental age.

Finally, in regard to motor learning-control processes, it has been reported that individuals with Down syndrome have deficits in short-term memory, storage and retrieval, particularly in relation to visual stimuli (Bouffard, 1990; McDade and Adler, 1980). Deficiencies have also been reported in the motor control of individuals with Down syndrome, especially in timing of movements (Block, 1991; Davis, Sparrow and Ward, 1991; Henderson and Hall, 1982) (see Chapter 6 for a review of the motor control literature).

The evidence from the previous section indicates that persons with Down syndrome have advanced processing deficiencies which together with deficiencies in basic and intermediate processes will affect their motor development.

CONCLUSIONS AND IMPLICATIONS FOR THE BOOK FROM THIS OVERVIEW OF ABNORMAL MOTOR DEVELOPMENT

From this review of literature it is evident that children who are clumsy or intellectually disabled and children with Down syndrome have deficiencies in sensory-neurological, integrative-perceptual and motor learning-control processes but these deficiencies differ for each category of disability. For instance, clumsy children were reported to exhibit minor neurological abnormalities, achieve in motor performance tasks at a lower level than normal peers and have apparent problems in motor control, as indicated by their jerky, poorly timed movements and slower responses to complex movements. Intellectually disabled children were found to have delayed postural reflexes and delayed ability to process, integrate, store and retrieve sensory information, in fact in many of these areas their performance is closer to that of normally developing children of the same mental age, than children of the same chronological age. Children with Down syndrome have delayed reflex development, low muscle tone (hypotonia), slow movements, problems in integrating sensory information and in organizing a movement response, and controlling the force of their movements. Children with intellectual disability and Down syndrome have marked delays in their gross motor development.

It was not possible from the literature to gain a comprehensive picture of the motor problems for each of these categories of children. This is because most of the previous research has tended to assess children on only one aspect of motor development.

In subsequent chapters there is a review of relevant literature and a report on original studies, by the authors, into the motor performance, fundamental movement patterns and interlimb coordination of children who are clumsy or intellectually disabled or who have Down syndrome.

REFERENCES

Anastasiow, N.J. (1986) *Developmental and Disability*. Paul H. Brooks, Baltimore, London.

Bairstow, P.J. and Lazlo, I.J. (1981) Kinesthetic sensitivity to passive movements and its relationship to motor development and motor control. *Developmental Medicine and Child Neurology*, **23**, 606–16.

Berry, P., Gunn, V.P. and Andrews, R.J. (1984) Development of Down's Syndrome children from birth to five years. *Perspectives and Progress in Mental Retardation*, **1**, 167–77.

Block, M.E. (1991) Motor development in children with Down's Syndrome: a review of literature. *Adapted Physical Activity Quarterly*, **8**, 175–209.

Bouffard, M. (1990) Movement problem solutions by educable mentally handicapped individuals. *Adapted Physical Activity Quarterly*, **7**, 183–197.

Boulton-Lewis, G. and Catherwood, D. (1994) *The Early Years*. The Australian Council for Educational Research, Victoria, Australia.

Bruininks, R. (1978) *Bruininks–Oseretsky Test of Motor Proficiency: Examiners Manual*. American Guidance Services, Circle Pines, MN.

Bullock, M.I. and Watter, P. (1987) Patterns of motor development in children with minimal cerebral dysfunction, in *Tenth International Congress World Federation for Physical Therapy*, Sydney, Link Printing, pp. 280–4.

Butterworth, G. and Cicchetti, D. (1978) Visual calibration of posture in normal and motor retarded Down's Syndrome infants. *Perception*, **7**, 513–25.

Carr, J. (1992) Longitudinal research in Down Syndrome. *International Review of Research in Mental Retardation*, **18**, 197–223.

Chenoweth, R. and Bullock, M.I. (1978) A comparative study of the sensori-motor capacities of normal and intellectually handicapped children. *Australian Journal of Mental Retardation*, **5**, 20–5.

Crome, I., Cowie, V. and Slater, E. (1966) Statistical note on cerebellar and brain stem weight in mongolism. *Journal of Mental Deficiency*, **10**, 1969–72.

Davidson, P.W., Pine, R., Wiles-Kettenmann, M. and Appelle, S. (1980) Haptic-visual shape matching by mentally retarded children: explanatory activity and complexity effects. *American Journal of Mental Deficiency*, **84**, 526–33.

Davis, W.E. (1984) Motor ability assessment of populations with handicapping conditions: challenging basic assumptions. *Adapted Physical Activity Quarterly*, **1**, 125–40.

Davis, W.E. and Sinning, W.E. (1987) Muscle stiffness in Down Syndrome and other mentally handicapped subjects: a research note. *Journal of Motor Behaviour*, **19**, 130–44.

Davis, W.E., Sparrow, W.A. and Ward, T. (1991) Fractional reaction times and movement times of Down's Syndrome and other adults with mental retardation. *Adapted Physical Activity Quarterly*, **8**, 221–33.

Dyer, S., Gunn, P., Rauh, H. and Berry, P. (1990) Motor development in Down Syndrome children: an analysis of the motor scale of the Bayley Scales of Infant Development, in *Motor Development in Children: Aspects of Coordination and Control*, (eds M.G. Wade and H.T.A. Whiting), Martinus Nijhoff, Dordrecht, pp. 107–21.

Fischer, K.W. and Farrar, M.J. (1988) Generalizations about generalizations: how a theory of skill development explains both generality and specificy, in *The Neo-Piagetian Theories of Cognitive Development: Towards an Integration*, (ed. A. Demetriou), North-Holland, Elsevier, Amsterdam, pp. 137–71.

Fischer, K.W. and Lazerson, A. (1984) *Human Development*, Freeman, New York.

Fischer, K.W. and Silvern, L.E. (1985) Stages and individual difference in cognitive development. *Annual Review of Psychology*, **36**, 613–48.

Geuze, R. and Borger, H. (1993) Children who are clumsy: five years later. *Adapted Physical Activity Quarterly*, **10**, 10–21.

Geuze, R.H. and Kalverboer, A.F. (1987) Inconsistency and adaptation in timing of clumsy children. *Journal of Human Movement Studies*, **13**, 421–3.

Gillberg, I.C. (1985) Children with minor neurodevelopmental disorders: neurological and neurodevelopmental problems at age 10. *Developmental Medicine and Child Neurology*, **27**, 3–16.

Gillberg, I.C., Gillbert, C. and Groth, J. (1989) Children with preschool minor neurodevelopmental disorders, V: neurodevelopmental profiles at age 13. *Developmental Medicine and Child Neurology*, **31**, 16–24.

Gordon, N. and McKinlay, I. (eds) (1980) *Helping Clumsy Children*. Churchill Livingstone, Edinburgh.

Gubbay, S. (1975) *The Clumsy Child*, W.B. Saunders, London.

Gubbay, S. (1978) The management of developmental apraxia. *Developmental Medicine and Child Neurology*, **20**, 643–6.

Gubbay, S. (1989) The clumsy child. *Modern Medicine of Australia*. November, 14–19.

Haley, S.M. (1986) Postural reactions in infants with Down Syndrome: relationship to motor milestone development and age. *Physical Therapy*, **66**, 17–22.

Hallam, P., Weindling, A.M., Klenka, H. *et al*. (1993) A comparison of three procedures to assess the motor ability of 12-month-old infants with cerebral palsy. *Developmental Medicine and Child Neurology*, **35**, 602–7.

Halverson, L.E., Roberton, M.A. and Langendorfer, S. (1982) Development of the overarm throw: movement and ball velocity changes by seventh grade. *Research Quarterly for Exercise and Sport*, **53**, 198–205.

Hardin, D.H. and Garcia, M.J. (1982) Diagnostic performance tests for elementary school children (grades 1–4). *Journal of Physical Education Recreation and Dance*, **53**, 48–9.

Harris, S.R. (1981) Effects of neurodevelopmental therapy on motor performance of infants with Down's Syndrome. *Developmental Medicine and Child Neurology*, **23**, 477–83.

Hayes, A. (1990) Developmental psychology, education and the need to move beyond typological thinking. *Australian Journal of Education*, **34**, 235–41.

Hayes, A. and Gunn, P. (1991) Developmental assumptions about Down's syndrome and the myth of uniformity, in *Adolescents with Down Syndrome: International Perspectives on Research and Program Development*, (ed. C.J. Denholm), University of Victoria, Victoria, BC, pp. 73–81.

Hellegren, L., Gillberg, C. Gillberg, I.C. and Enerskog, I. (1993) Children with deficits in attention, motor control and perception

(DAMP) almost grown up: general health at 16 years of age. *Developmental Medicine and Child Neurology*, **35**, 881–92.

Henderson, S.E. (1985) Motor skill development, in *Current Approaches to Down's Syndrome*, (eds D. Lane and B. Stratford), Holt, Rinehart & Winston, London, pp. 187–213.

Henderson, S.E. (1987) The assessment of clumsy children: old and new approaches. *Journal of Child Psychology and Psychiatry*, **28**, 511–29.

Henderson, S.E. and Hall, D. (1982) Concomitants of clumsiness in young school children. *Developmental Medicine and Child Neurology*, **24**, 448–60.

Henderson, S.E., Knight, E. Losse, A. and Jongmans, M. (1991) The clumsy child in school – are we doing enough? *British Journal of Physical Education: Research Supplement*, **9**, 2–7.

Hoare, D. and Larkin, D. (1991) Kinesthetic abilities of clumsy children. *Developmental Medicine and Child Neurology*, **33**, 671–8.

Hoover, J.H. and Wade, M.G. (1985) Motor learning theory. *Adapted Physical Activity Quarterly*, **2**, 228–52.

Hulme, C., Biggerstaff, A., Moran, G. and McKinlay, I. (1982) Visual, kinaesthetic and cross-modal judgements of length by normal and clumsy children. *Developmental Medicine and Child Neurology*, **24**, 461–71.

Kirk, S.A. and Gallagher, J.J. (1986) *Educating Exceptional Children*. Houghton Mifflin, Boston.

Larkin, D. and Hoare, D. (1991) *Out of Step*. The University of Western Australia, Nedlands.

Larkin, D. and Hoare, D. (1992) The movement approach: a window to understanding the clumsy child, *Approaches to The Study of Motor Control and Learning*, (ed. J.J. Summers), North Holland, Elsevier Science, Amsterdam, pp. 413–40.

Lazarus, J.C. and Todor, J.I. (1991) The role of attention in the regulation of associated movement in children. *Developmental Medicine and Child Neurology*, **33**, 32–9.

Lazlo, J.I. and Bairstow, P.J. (1985) *Perceptual-Motor Behaviour: Developmental Assessment and Therapy*. Holt, Rinehart & Winston, London.

Lazlo, J.I. Bartrip, J. and Rolfe, U. (1988) Clumsiness or perceptuo-motor dysfunction? in *Cognition and Action in Skilled Behaviour*, (eds A.M. Colley and J.R. Beech), Elsevier, Amsterdam, pp. 293–310.

Lincoln, A.J., Courchene, E., Kilman, B.A. and Galambos, R. (1985) Neuropsychological correlates of information-processing by children with Down Syndrome. *American Journal of Mental Deficiency*, **4**, 403–14.

Losse, A., Henderson, S.E., Elliman, D. *et al.* (1991) Clumsiness in children do they grow out of it? a ten year follow-up study. *Developmental Medicine and Child Neurology*, **33**, 55–69.

Lydic, J.S. and Steele, C. (1979) Assessment of the quality of sitting and gait patterns in children with Down's Syndrome. *Physical Therapy*, **59**, 1489–94.

Maeland, A.F. (1992) Identification of children with motor co-ordination problems. *Adapted Physical Activity Quarterly*, **9**, 330–42.

Marchiori, G.E., Wall, A.E. and Bedingfield, W. (1987) Kinematic analysis of skill acquisition in physically awkward boys. *Adapted Physical Activity Quarterly*, **3**, 305–15.

McCarron, L.T. (1982) *MAND McCarron Assessment of Neuromuscular Development*, rev. edn. Common Market Press, Dallas.

McDade, H.L. and Adler, S. (1980) Down syndrome and short-term memory impairment: a storage or retrieval deficit. *American Journal of Mental Deficiency*, **84**, 561–7.

McKinlay, I. (1980) Why are they clumsy? in *Helping Clumsy Children* (eds N. Gordon and I. McKinlay) Churchill Livingstone, Edinburgh.

Molnar, G.E. (1978) Analysis of motor disorder in retarded infants and young children. *American Journal of Mental Deficiency*, **83**, 213–22.

Newell, K.M. and Barclay, C.R. (1982) Developing knowledge about action, in *The Development of Movement Control and Co-ordination* (eds J.A.S. Kelso and J.E. Clark), John Wiley, Chichester, pp. 175–212.

O'Brien, C.C. (1988) Motor development in clumsy, intellectually disabled and Down's syndrome children; a comparative study. Unpublished PhD Thesis, University of Queensland.

O'Brien, C.C. and Hayes, A. (1989) Motor development in early childhood of clumsy, intellectually disabled and Down's Syndrome children. *The ACHPER National Journal*, **124**, 15–19.

Parker, A.W., Bronks, R. and Snyder, C.W. (1986) Walking patterns in Down's Syndrome. *Journal of Mental Deficiency Research*, **30**, 317–30.

Parker, A.W. and James, B. (1985) Age changes in the flexibility of Down's Syndrome children. *Journal of Mental Deficiency Research*, **29**, 207–18.

Rarick, G.L. (1981) The emergence of the study of human motor development, in *Perspectives on the Academic Discipline of Physical Education*, (ed. G.A. Brooks), Human Kinetics, Champaign, IL, pp. 163–89.

Rarick, G.L. (1982) Descriptive research and process-oriented explanations of the motor development of children, in *The Development of Movement Control and Co-ordination*, (eds J.A.S. Kelso and J.E. Clark), John Wiley, Chichester, pp. 275–91.

Rasmussen, P., Gillberg, C., Waldenstrom, E. and Svenson, B. (1983) Perceptual, motor and attentional deficits in seven-year-old children: neurological and neurodevelopmental aspects. *Developmental Medicine and Child Neurology*, **25**, 315–33.

Rast, M.M. and Harris, S.A. (1985) Motor control in infants with Down's Syndrome. *Developmental Medicine and Child Neurology*, **27**, 675–85.

Reid, G. (1985) Physical activity programming, in *Current Approaches*

to Down's Syndrome, (eds D. Lane and B. Stratford), Holt, Rinehart & Winston, London, pp. 219–41.
Share, J. and French, R. (1982) *Motor Development of Down's Syndrome Children: Birth to 6 Years*. US Department of Education, National Institute of Education Research.
Shepherd, R.B. (1980) Problem analysis with Down's Syndrome infants. *Cumberland College Reports*, **20**, 1–14.
Sherrill, C. (1986) *Adapted Pysical Education and Recreation*, Wm. C. Brown, Dubuque, IA.
Shumway-Cook, A. and Woollacott, M.H. (1988) Dynamics of postural control in the child with Down's Syndrome. *Physical Therapy*, **65**, 1315–22.
Smyth, M.M. (1986) Relating cognition and action: reaction to Mounoud, in *Motor Development in Children: Aspects of Coordination and Control* (eds M.G. Wade and H.T.A. Whiting), Martinus Nijhoff, Dordretch, pp. 391–403.
Smyth, T.R. (1991) Abnormal clumsiness in children: a defect of motor programming? *Child Care Health and Development*, **17**, 283–94.
Smyth, T.R. (1992) Impaired motor skill (clumsiness) in otherwise normal children: a review. *Child Care, Health and Development*, **18**, 283–300.
Thelen, E. (1986) Development of coordinated movement: implications for early movement development, in *Motor Development in Children: Aspects of Coordination and Control*, (eds M.G. Wade and H.T.A. Whiting), Martinus Nijhoff, Dordretch, pp. 107–21.
Thomas, J.R. (1984) Children's motor skill development, in *Motor Development During Childhood and Adolescence*, Burgess, Minneapolis, pp. 91–104.
Thombs, B. and Sugden, D. (1991) Manual skills in Down Syndrome children ages 6–16 years. *Adapted Physical Activity Quarterly*, **8**, 242–52.
Touwen, B. (1990) Development of the brain in mentally deficient children: conceptual considerations, in *Motor Development, Adapted Physical Activity and Mental Retardation*, Vol. 30, (ed A. Vermeer), Karger, Basle, pp. 1–6.
van Dellen, T. and Geuze, R.H. (1988) Motor response processing in clumsy children. *Journal of Child Psychology and Psychiatry*, **29**, 489–500.
van der Meulen, J.H.P., Denier van der Gon, J.J., Gielen, C.C.A.M. and Willemse, J. (1991) Visuomotor performance of normal and clumsy children. 1: Fast goal-directed arm-movements with and without visual feedback. *Developmental Medicine and Child Neurology*, **33**, 40–54.
Wickstrom, R.L. (1983) Fundamental motor patterns, Lea & Febiger, Philadelphia.
Williams, H.G., Woollacott, M.H. and Ivry, R.(1992) Timing and control in clumsy children. *Journal of Motor Behavior*, **24**, 165–72.
Woollacott, M.H. (1993) Normal and abnormal development of posture control in children. Paper presented at *The 9th International*

Symposium on Adapted Physical Activity, Yokohama, Japan, August, 1993.

Zelaznick, H.N. (1986) Issues in the study of human motor skill development: a reaction to John Fentress, in *Motor Development in Children: Aspects of Coordination and Control*, (eds M.G. Wade and H.T.A. Whiting), Martinus Nijhoff, Dordrecht, pp. 107–21.

Zigler, E. and Hodapp, R.M. (1986) *Understanding Mental Retardation*, Cambridge University Press, Cambridge.

3

Motor performance

The aim of this chapter is to examine motor performance in normally developing and motor impaired children. Motor performance is the first aspect of movement behaviour to be investigated. It is the basis for inferences about the level of skill that has been acquired and is an aspect of movement behaviour that can be measured quantitatively. As already indicated, motor performance scores also reflect the influence of maturation, experience, motor learning and motor control. In a review of changes in motor skills during childhood, however, Branta, Haubenstricker and Seefeldt (1984, p. 467) made the pertinent comment that describing and explaining the postural and locomotor adjustments of humans during the course of their adaptations to a changing structure is an awesome task.

This chapter consists of a literature review that examines the factors affecting motor performance and the changes in motor skills and performance in early and middle childhood, for each of the three categories of motor impaired children that are the focus of this volume. The final section of the chapter reports and discusses results of a study conducted by the authors to determine the differences in motor performance levels between normally developing and motor impaired children.

OVERVIEW

Various methodological problems are encountered when attempting to study changes in motor performance, for example, many of the studies use different administration techniques for similar motor tasks. Despite such methodological problems, studies measuring motor performance have provided knowledge about what children and adults can be expected to achieve, and allow statements to be made about children's level of performance on complex skills. Nevertheless, such measures merely document changes in performance scores and do not provide a basis for explaining how and why the changes occur. In short they provide information about motor products but little information about the processes underlying motor performance.

Notwithstanding, standardized motor performance tests are useful because they provide normative data against which individual and group performance can be compared. Such information also enables decisions to be made in regard to whether a child is developing normally or differently. Motor performance tests are also generally norm-referenced so allowing comparison to be made between the motor performance of normally developing children and between these children and motor impaired children.

Before describing an example of a study to investigate similarities and differences between normal and motor impaired children relevant literature on their motor behaviour will be reviewed. The progression of motor performance in normally developing children is examined first, then the pattern of progression will be examined for clumsy and intellectually disabled children and children with Down syndrome.

NORMALLY DEVELOPING CHILDREN

Factors affecting motor performance in normally developing children

Factors which are likely to influence motor performance in children include the neural and reflex substrates, growth, maturation and cognitive processes (Smoll, 1982). The factors affecting change in motor performance, in early and middle childhood, to be addressed in this section include physical changes, such as growth and changes related to gender (Hills, 1991; Malina, 1974, 1981, 1984). The sensory-neurological, integrative-perceptual, motor learning-control processes have been discussed in Chapter 1. Some of the physical changes that occur with increased age are quantitative, such as increase in body size particularly in terms of height, weight and strength. Of these changes stature, leg length and fat distribution in a child, are more likely to be influenced by inheritance than body weight and bone dimensions, which are more dependent on environmental influences (Malina, 1984).

Increase in size does not proceed at a constant rate, for instance gain in weight is almost twice as great as gain in height, and lower limbs grow more rapidly than the trunk. Additionally, the rate of gain in height and weight from one phase in childhood to another varies. For example, the gain is rapid in infancy and early childhood, with a slower growth rate in middle childhood (Malina, 1984). There are also gender-related differences. For example, males tend to be taller and heavier at all ages, and although the rate of growth in both is similar to that of females in early and middle childhood, girls have longer legs compared with their trunk length than boys of the same chronological age, until puberty (Espenchade and Eckert, 1980; Hills, 1991).

Together with an age-related increase in height there is also an increase in strength which is greatest in boys from 7 years of age (Rarick, 1981), but reaches its peak at about 9–10 years, in girls, and 11–12 years of age in boys (Espenchade and Eckert, 1980; Malina, 1984). Weight gain, which is another component in the changes in body size of children, is dependent on changes in different tissues at different ages. The rapid growth rate in early childhood plays a role in weight gain because growth and ossification of bone are a major contribution to weight increase. Moreover, up to five years of age muscle tissue changes represent 25% of total body weight. By the sixth year, however, muscle tissue comprises 75% of weight gained (Espenchade and Eckert, 1980; Hills, 1991).

Body build or physique is another factor that may contribute to changes in motor performance, it incorporates stature, weight, and muscle size. The child's motor performance is more highly correlated with physique, in early childhood than in middle childhood. The heavily muscled (mesomorphic) type of body build gives children a performance advantage because these children have greater muscular strength than children who have lower muscle strength and more fat tissue (endomorphic build). There also is a tendency for gender differences, in that more girls have an endomorphic physique and more boys have a mesomorphic physique (Hills, 1991; Malina, 1974).

The contributions of body stature, and physique to changes in motor performance have been subjected to considerable scrutiny in the last 20 years. In regard to changes in physique, for example, Malina (1974) stated that there is evidence in early childhood that children with higher than normal subcutaneous fat do not perform as well as children with less fat, on running and jumping tasks. The correlation between body build and motor performance in middle childhood, however, is only affected by extremes in body configuration (Malina, 1974, 1984). Despite this claim there is still a tendency in both age groups for endomorphic children to perform at lower levels on motor tasks where the body is projected (such as in running and jumping), than mesomorphic and ectomorphic peers. Conversely, when the motor skill incorporates throwing an object, such as a ball, there is a positive correlation with larger body size and physique (Malina, 1984). Nevertheless, the commonly held belief that larger children for their age are more likely to be superior in motor skills has been disputed, because an increase in body height and weight results in increased inertia of the body, so in order to maintain or improve physical performance there must be a correspondingly greater increase in strength (Newell, 1984).

Another factor which has received considerable attention in the literature, is the difference in motor performance between boys and girls. There is evidence which shows that boys are superior in running, jumping and throwing activities whereas girls are superior in activities such as hopping and skipping (Broadhead and Church, 1985; De Oreo, 1974; Morris *et al.*, 1982). These differences appear in early childhood and continue throughout life. Nevertheless, other researchers have found that although there is a significant difference between the mean scores of boys and girls, the distributions overlap, and many girls performed motor skills just as well as boys, particularly when comparing boys and girls of similar physique (Espenchade and Eckert, 1980; Rarick, 1981).

In summary, motor performance in early and middle childhood is influenced by factors related to physical growth and gender. The patterns of change that have been documented in various skills, in normally developing children, will be discussed in the next section.

Motor performance in normally developing children

Rapid growth and motor development in children peaks at approximately 4–5 years of age. The literature on motor performance, in early childhood, has revealed that chronological age is an important indicator of improvement in motor tasks (e.g., Broadhead and Church, 1985; Erbaugh, 1984; Morris *et al.*, 1982; O'Brien, 1988). Motor performance in normally developing children improves and variability in performance increases as children grow older (Branta, Haubenstricker and Seefeldt, 1984).

Branta *et al.* (1984) summarized the results of a 16-year longitudinal study on motor performance. The means and standard deviations were derived from two age groupings (5–10 and 8–14 year olds). It was reported that, with the exception of the flexibility task, there was an age-related improvement in tasks which measured leg power, such as jump and reach and standing long jump. In the 30 yards' dash, 120 feet agility run and the 400 feet shuttle run there was a rapid improvement in speed from ages 5 to 7 years followed by steady improvement until about age 14 years. The authors reported little gender-related difference in performance except that boys were superior in the flexed arm hang test from 7 years of age, and girls were consistently more flexible in the sit and reach tasks at all ages (Branta *et al.*, 1984).

The trend for age-related improvement in motor performance in children alters at about 13 years of age. In girls, improvement in many motor tasks tends to slow down, whereas boys continue to improve in many tasks until about 18 years of age (Branta *et al.*, 1984; Espenchade and Eckert, 1980). It should be noted, however, that the reported superiority of boys' motor performance often has not been supported by statistically significant results (Branta *et al.*, 1984).

As stated previously, improvement in motor performance with increased chronological age is often assumed to be due to age-related increases in strength, height and weight in children. Recently doubts have been cast on such assumptions. For example, in middle childhood, motor performance only seems to be affected at the extremes of height, weight and physique. An alternative explanation for the improvement and differences in performance in motor skills in older children is that factors like practice and motivation play an increasingly important part (Espenchade and Eckert, 1980).

This section has summarized current knowledge about factors that contribute to changes in motor performance of normally developing children. It provides the basis for a comparison of motor performance among groups of clumsy, intellectually disabled and children with Down syndrome. The majority of these children have motor performance scores below normally developing age peers. Factors which affect motor performance and changes in motor performance with increased age in these groups of motor impaired children will be reviewed in the following sections. First, motor performance in clumsy children will be discussed, followed by an examination of data from children with intellectually disability or Down syndrome.

CLUMSY CHILDREN

Factors affecting motor performance in clumsy children

It has been reported that on physical examination, there was no difference in height, weight or head circumference between children of normal intelligence with normal motor development and those who were designated as clumsy (Gubbay, 1975; Lockwood, 1987). Despite this claim, a recent study has demonstrated a significant difference between the somatotype of well-coordinated and age-matched clumsy children (Hoare and Larkin, 1991). More of the clumsy children were of endomorphic body type which is characterized by an increase in fat tissue in comparison with muscle tissue. It is feasible that both an increase in fat tissue and a decrease in strength, as well as the sensory-neurological, integrative-perceptual and motor learning-control deficits of clumsy children, make it more difficult for them to perform motor skills. Nevertheless, the major finding in clumsy children from approximately 4 years of age is an ineptitude in motor performance and/or below age standards in motor skills and motor tasks (Henderson, 1987; Henderson and Hall, 1982; Hoare and Larkin, 1991; Larkin and

Hoare, 1991, 1992; O'Brien and Hayes, 1989). For this reason the criterion of motor skills at a level below normal for age is used to identify clumsy children in this book.

Motor performance in clumsy children

Reports by parents, teachers, and children on their ability at sport do not correlate highly with diagnosed developmental clumsiness (Gubbay, 1975). Similarly, a study by Keogh *et al.* (1979) found that there was no correlation between observational ratings of physical skills in primary school children by classroom teachers and trained physical education teachers. A later study, however, showed that a check-list on physical competence filled out by classroom teachers, was reliable in terms of identifying children with the more severe coordination problems, as determined by the TOMI test (Stott, Henderson and Moyes, 1986).

Additionally, another study reported that children in infants schools who were rated as clumsy by classroom teachers did have difficulty with static and dynamic balance, ball skills, manual dexterity, gross motor control and production of simultaneous movements (Henderson and Hall, 1982). These authors noted, however, that only five of 16 children selected by teachers for their study could be classified as having an isolated gross motor disability, whereas in the remaining clumsy children motor impairment was only one of many disabilities. This latter finding is in agreement with the work of other researchers (e.g. Bullock and Watter, 1987; Gillberg, 1985; Henderson, 1985, 1987; Losse *et al.*, 1991; Paine, Werry and Quay, 1968).

In summary, there is evidence that clumsy children perform on motor tasks and motor skills below normal for their chronological age. This factor alone, points to the need for further studies on clumsy children, in order to understand the problems which they experience in motor development and, additionally, to collect data on their patterns of developmental change.

INTELLECTUALLY DISABLED CHILDREN

Factors affecting motor performance in intellectually disabled children

Children whose intellectual disability is not caused by genetic anomalies usually have been disabled by causes such as birth, trauma, prematurity, infection, metabolic imbalance and nutritional disorders. In many cases the cause is unknown. One result of intellectual disability is an increased likelihood of problems in movement coordination. Such problems may hinder acquisition of complex skills and consequently affect levels of motor performance.

Unlike the low association between scores on intelligence tests and motor performance tests in normally developing children, this situation is reversed for motor performance in intellectually disabled children. Indeed, the more severe the intellectual disability, the lower the level of performance on motor tasks (Rarick, 1981). Undoubtedly, some of this performance lag can be attributed to factors which also affect the child's overall development, including body size, strength and neurological factors.

Apart from those children who have chromosome or metabolic disorders, most mildly intellectually disabled children are hard to distinguish from their normal peers in terms of stature (Rarick, Dobbins and Broadhead, 1976; Sherrill, 1986). Nevertheless, as a group these children are heavier in relationship to their height than normal children (Rarick, Dobbins and Broadhead, 1976). Skinfold tests have shown that the extra weight is caused by excessive adipose (fat) tissue. This excess fat tissue is probably due to the fact that mildly intellectually disabled children have been shown to have lower activity levels than normal children (Lockwood, 1987; Rarick, Dobbins and Broadhead, 1976).

In tests of strength and explosive muscle force it has been shown that mildly intellectually disabled boys and girls aged 6–9 years and 10–13 years of age have measures on these factors, similar to those of normally developing children aged between 2 and 4 years younger (Rarick, Dobbins and Broadhead, 1976). This deficit together with the tendency for increased weight for height hinders performance on tasks requiring explosive muscular force such as running, jumping and throwing a ball for speed and distance. In addition, they are generally muscularly and physically unfit (Cratty, 1979, Winnick and Short, 1991).

The reviewed literature suggests that the main difference between normally developing and mildly intellectually disabled children is in the level achieved in motor performance tests, rather than in major differences in how motor tasks are performed (Connolly and Michael, 1986). Nevertheless, the factors affecting performance on these tests were found to be the same as for normally developing children. They were upper extremity coordination, rhythmic ability, general muscular coordination, gross motor functioning, praxis, dynamic balance, maturation and gender (Liemohn and Knapczyk, 1974).

Altogether, the evidence demonstrates that intellectually disabled chldren have many factors which tend to hinder or delay their motor performance. Whether children with Down syndrome have similar factors which affect their motor performance, or whether as an indentifiably different group they have specific factors typical of their impairment will be discussed in the section on motor performance of children with Down syndrome.

Motor performance in intellectually disabled children

The majority of children who are classified as mildly to moderately intellectually disabled (excluding those with diagnosed cerebral palsy), have been found to exhibit poor coordination in gross and fine motor skills and in locomotor patterns (Kirk and Gallagher, 1986). Sensory-neurological processes, in particular, affect their motor development. Indeed young intellectually disabled children have minor to marked delays in attaining upright locomotion. Some severely intellectually handicapped children, for example, do not walk until 7 years of age (Donoghue *et al.*, 1970). These delays have been attributed to slower maturation of the automatic postural mechanisms in intellectually disabled infants, who showed no other signs on a neurological examination of abnormalities in muscle tone, posture or involuntary movement (Molnar, 1978; Woollacott, 1993).

Children classified as intellectually disabled have been consistently reported as having lower motor performance levels than their intellectually normal peers (Connolly and Michael, 1986). Francis and Rarick (1959), for example, conducted a battery of motor performance tests on 284 intellectually disabled children (IQ scores ranged between 50 and 90), aged between 7 years 6 months and 14 years 6 months. The tests were designed to measure strength, power, balance and agility. Results were compared with available normative data and this showed that delay in motor performance varied from 6 years delay in 14-year-old intellectually disabled children (of either gender), in the standing broad jump, to 4 years delay in running speed and 1–3 years delay in many of the tests that measured strength. Francis and Rarick (1959) concluded from these data that intellectually disabled children obtained lower scores in all motor performance tasks, a trend which becomes greater with increased age.

The severity of motor impairment in intellectually disabled children has also been recorded by Dobbins and Rarick (1976) who found that the motor performance of approximately 14% of mildly intellectually disabled boys could not be distinguished from about 93% of intellectually normal boys, whereas only 9.8% of intellectually normal boys could not be distinguished from the intellectually disabled boys (mean age 8 years 6 months, age range 6 years 0 months to 9 years 9 months). Similar trends were reported by Rarick (1981, 1982) who claimed that the average motor performance of mildly intellectually disabled boys was lower than 87% of normal age peers, and that 95% of mildly intellectually disabled girls had motor performance scores lower than their normally developing peers.

A further study compared the ability of intellectually disabled children to balance on a stabiliometer (Eckert and Rarick, 1976). Children were divided into three groups (mildly intellectually disabled aged 6–9 years and 10–13 years; and normal children aged 6–9 years). The normal children served as the comparison group since they were the same chronological age as the younger mildly intellectually disabled children and the same mental age as the older mildly intellectually disabled children. It was found that normal children had a higher performance score than mildly intellectually disabled children of the same age, and that the older children actually had a lower performance than the younger intellectually disabled children.

In conclusion, the studies that have been described on motor performance in mildly intellectually disabled children indicate that as a group these children obtain lower scores in motor performance tasks, and have lower general motor ability than their intellectually normal peers. For further studies on motor performance of intellectually disabled children, see those of Henderson, Morris and Ray (1981) and Connolly and Michael (1986). Both studies compare the results of intellectually disabled children, with and without Down syndrome, and their performance scores on a gross motor test. They are reviewed in the next section.

CHILDREN WITH DOWN SYNDROME

Factors affecting motor performance in children with Down syndrome

The chromosomal abnormality resulting in Down syndrome, causes many deviations in physical growth and posture in these children (Chapter 2). For example, they generally have a short stature, primarily caused by reduced length of the lower extremities in relation to the rest of their body (Barden, 1985). This delay in growth is evident from birth when they are already shorter in stature and weigh less than normal infants. It has been reported that by three years of age children with Down syndrome are more than two standard deviations below normal stature and have increased weight for their length, when compared with normal children (Cronk, 1978; Cronk, Chumlea and Roche, 1985). Moreover, the growth rates for length and weight are different from that of normal children. Under two years of age the rates are below those of normal children, but there is evidence which indicates that from 4 years of age children with Down syndrome grow at the same rate as normal children (Barden, 1985; Cronk, 1978; Malina, 1981).

Children with Down syndrome usually have postural mechanism deficits likely to affect motor performance (Woollacott, 1993). They also have postural problems, frequently in the vertebral column, which results in conditions such as atlanto-axial subluxation of the cervical region (Cooke, 1984; Semine *et al.*, 1978). In addition, many of these children have deformities in the lower extremities, such as external tibial torsion, pes valgus, recurrent dislocation of the patella and congenitally dislocated hips (Mahan, Diamond and Brown, 1983). Many of these postural abnormalities, together with the abnormal sitting and walking postures, have been attributed to lax ligaments and hypermobility of the joints (Lydic and Steele, 1979; Parker and James, 1985). It is feasible that the generalized low muscle tone evident from birth in over 97% of children with Down syndrome (McIntire and Dutch, 1964) also contributes to their abnormal posture and postural development.

Low muscle tone (hypertonia) is another dominant characteristic of the physical development of children with Down syndrome. Morris, Vaughan and Vaccaro (1982) conducted a study to measure muscle tone and strength changes in children with Down syndrome ($n=28$; ages 4–6 years, 9–11 years, and 12–15+ years), who were compared with normal subjects ($n=33$, ages 4–17 years). The patella reflex response was measured in an attempt to quantify changes, and differences, in muscle tone. A hand dynamometer was used to measure differences in strength between the two groups. The authors' findings were that there was a significant difference between both groups, with the normally developing children demonstrating greater muscle tone and strength. However, they found a slight increase in muscle tone in the older age group with Down syndrome which suggested some improvement in tone with increased age. They argued that this improvement may be related to increased muscle strength in the older children with Down syndrome.

As well as sensory-neurological deficits, integrative-perceptual processes affecting motor performance have been reported in the literature. Kerr and Blais (1985), for example, found that the children with Down syndrome were slower in their reactions on a visual-tracking task but were more accurate than other (non-Down syndrome) intellectually disabled peers. It is possible that decreased ability to predict direction on a tracking task could be due to deficits in visual-motor coordination in people with Down syndrome. Additionally, the slower speed in their visual-tracking response, when compared with normal and intellectually disabled subjects, could be related to their low muscle tone and to their lower intellectual ability. Both these factors would affect their motor performance in tasks such as catching a ball.

From the previous discussion it is apparent that physical factors have far-reaching effects on the motor performance capabilities of children with Down syndrome. They appear, as a group of children, to be at the extremely low end of the distribution for height and strength, while at the very high end for weight. Moreover, both hypotonia, poor balance mechanisms and visual–motor coordination are factors likely to contribute to the lower motor performance that has been reported in these children.

Motor performance in children with Down syndrome

According to Henderson (1985) children with Down syndrome seem to acquire and perform motor skills at older ages than their peers but with increased age they tend to become more disabled in motor development than normally developing children. She noted, however, that there is a great deal of variability in their motor development. Further evidence of delayed motor development in children with Down syndrome, is that they have been shown to perform most motor tasks at a level which is about 2 years behind their normal peers. This trend of delay in performance of motor tasks continues during middle childhood, particularly in tasks which involve laterality, balance and hand–eye coordination (Dyer *et al.*, 1990; Share and French, 1982).

The discrepancy in motor task performance, however, is greatest in adults with Down syndrome, who seem to have difficulty in performing even simple motor tasks. Kerr and Blais (1985), for example, found that when 18-year-old subjects with Down syndrome were tested on a visual tracking task, they were not able to predict probable direction in the same way as normally developing and intellectually disabled individuals of the same age. In fact, their performance on these tasks was similar to children who had the same functional age (namely 7 years 6 months). Similar results, however, may not apply to younger children with Down syndrome, as many younger children have received early intervention, which would not have been widely available when Kerr and Blais's subjects were children.

Studies of motor performance of children with Down syndrome compared to other groups of children in motor performance tests have reported conflicting results. Le Blanc, French, and Schultz (1977), for instance, investigated Cratty's unpublished report that children with intellectual disability or Down syndrome were less proficient in the static and dynamic balance tasks on his Six Category Gross Motor Test than other moderately intellectually disabled children. Their results, for children with Down syndrome or intellectual disability aged 12 years (mean age = 12 years 3 months, IQ = 39.72) were contrary to those of Cratty. Specifically, these researchers found that children with Down syndrome were not significantly different from the other intellectually disabled children in the static balance tests, but were significantly better than the other children in the dynamic balance tasks.

A study conducted by Henderson, Morris and Ray (1981) compared the motor performance of children with Down syndrome or intellectual disability, matched for mental and chronological age, on the Cratty Gross Motor Test. The children were aged between 7 and 14 years. The results revealed variability in performance and some overlap between the groups. Altogether, children with Down syndrome performed tasks more slowly, balance tasks appeared more difficult for them, and their overall results were lower than the intellectually disabled control group. The only significant difference between the groups, however, was that intellectually disabled subjects were better than children with Down syndrome in the gross motor agility and locomotor agility tasks, both of which required postural changes of the body.

The performance on the Bruininks–Oseretsky Test of Motor Proficiency of intellectually disabled children, with and without Down syndrome, was investigated by Connolly and Michael (1986). The ages of the children with Down syndrome ranged from 7 years 7 months to 10 years 6 months (mean = 9 years 2 months) and the intellectually disabled children were aged between 7 years 11 months and 11 years (mean = 10 years 2 months). For both groups IQ scores were similar. The range for children with Down syndrome was 38–69 (mean = 54.5), and for the intellectually disabled children, 42–66 (mean = 56.8). In short all children were within the mild to moderate category of intellectual disability.

The authors reported that when tested on the subtests of running speed and agility, strength, visual–motor control, upper limb speed and dexterity and balance, children with Down syndrome performed at a significantly lower level than children with similar intellectual disability (Connolly and Michael, 1986). They were also significantly lower in their fine motor and gross motor composite scores. There were no significant differences between the groups on subtests dealing with bilateral coordination, upper limb coordination and response time.

To conclude this section, more studies are needed which investigate the motor performance of intellectually disabled and Down syndrome children. The reported studies suggest that their motor performance is below what would be expected of normally developing children of the same age. Nevertheless, studies using the Bruininks–Oseretsky Test, and Cratty's Gross Motor Test have not reported consistent findings.

SUMMARY OF FINDINGS FROM THE LITERATURE REVIEW ON MOTOR PERFORMANCE IN CHILDREN WHO ARE NORMALLY DEVELOPING, CLUMSY, INTELLECTUALLY DISABLED AND WITH DOWN SYNDROME

Several conclusions emerge from the literature review on factors affecting motor performance in children who are normally developing, clumsy, intellectually disabled or have Down syndrome. These are as follows:

1. It is only at either extreme of the continuum in terms of height and weight that motor performance in children is affected.
2. Strength, power and gross body coordination contribute the most to age-related changes in motor performance in normally developing children, in early and middle childhood. In middle childhood balance and rhythmical ability and ball skills are also important.
3. In normally developing children during early childhood, chronological age is more highly correlated with improvement in motor performance, than in middle childhood.
4. Differences in motor performance between boys and girls have been noted in early and middle childhood. Specifically, boys are usually superior in distance throwing, speed running, and standing long jump. Girls are generally better in tasks requiring bilateral body coordination such as skipping, balance (equivocal results) and fine motor tasks.

The reported gender differences have not always been verified statistically. Furthermore, when they have been verified the variability in children's individual performance is so large that the trend may not apply in individual cases. Girls and boys of the same physique also have similar motor performance scores.

5. There is some evidence to show that clumsy children of normal intelligence have a tendency to have more fat tissue and less muscular strength (i.e. an endomorphic physique), than their normal peers.
6. Mild to moderately intellectually disabled children have been shown to be heavier in relationship to their height than normally developing children. Children with Down syndrome are shorter, especially in distal limb segments, heavier, and have less strength than normal children of the same chronological age. For intellectually disabled children, and particularly for those with Down syndrome, anthropometric factors are likely to contribute in part to their documented poorer performance in motor tasks.
7. Clumsy children in early childhood have been identified on the basis of below age performance on static and dynamic balance, ball skills, manual dexterity, gross and fine motor control and production of simultaneous movements. The number of years they are behind their normally developing peers, in both early and middle childhood, is uncertain.
8. Mildly intellectually disabled children have been estimated as being 2–4 years behind chronological age norms in motor performance in all the conventional motor performance tasks. In addition, the gap between intellectually disabled and normal children seems to become greater with age.
9. It is estimated that children with Down syndrome are at least two years behind in terms of motor performance at 5 years of age and, as has been noted for intellectually disabled children, there is increased divergence from normally developing peers as they grow older.
10. Although the exact difference in motor performance, in comparison with normal and intellectually disabled children is uncertain, children with Down syndrome are reported to have consistently lower scores in most motor

tasks than intellectually disabled children with similar IQ scores. In one study using the Bruininks–Oseretsky Test of Motor Proficiency, Down syndrome children in middle childhood scored significantly lower than intellectually disabled cohorts in the subtests of running speed and agility, strength, visual motor control, upper limb speed, dexterity and balance, and in their fine motor and gross motor composite scores. No significant difference was found between the groups of children in subtests of bilateral coordination, upper limb coordination and response time.

11. Despite differences in rate of improvement, normally developing, clumsy, intellectually disabled and Down syndrome children all improve in performance of motor tasks with increased chronological age.

In conclusion, most of the studies reported in this literature review have compared the motor performance of normally developing and clumsy children, or of intellectually disabled and normally developing children of similar mental age, or the motor performance of children who are intellectually disabled and children with Down syndrome. No studies have been found which compare the motor performance of normally developing children with the three categories of motor impaired children of similar ages (namely clumsy, intellectually disabled and Down syndrome), hence, the study that is reported in the next section was conducted to rectify this situation.

A STUDY OF DIFFERENCES IN MOTOR PERFORMANCE IN CHILDREN WHO ARE NORMALLY DEVELOPING, CLUMSY, INTELLECTUALLY DISABLED AND WITH DOWN SYNDROME

A summary of the study by the authors comparing the motor performance of children who are normally developing, clumsy, intellectually disabled or with Down syndrome, will be reported in the next section. Differences among children with Down syndrome and intellectually disabled and clumsy children were examined by using items from an adapted version of the Bruininks–Oseretsky Test of Motor Proficiency (Bruininks, 1978). The short form (abbreviated BOT-S) of this test was chosen to assess the motor performance of the three categories of motor impaired children because it has been used previously on such populations and had been shown to provide a reasonable basis for describing the extent of motor delay in each of the motor impaired categories. (A review of the Bruininks–Oseretsky Test of Motor Proficiency and the adapted version of the BOT-S is given in Appendix A. Appendix A also includes the Method, Procedure and Results from the study.)

RESULTS, DISCUSSION AND IMPLICATIONS OF THE STUDY

The specific aims of the study were to determine first, whether motor impaired children performed at a lower level than normally developing children and second, whether any of the age groups and categories of children differed in terms of the rate or pattern of their performance as assessed by the test items. A final aim was to identify any areas in the performance of motor impaired children which might require specific attention in adapted motor programmes. (Appendix A, Part 1 gives more details on the characteristics of the motor impaired children who participated in the study. Also Appendix A, Part 2 consists of a summary of the literature related to the Bruininks–Oseretsky Test of Motor Proficiency.) The overall results from this cross-sectional study of the total raw scores and the five subtests of the adapted version of the Bruininks–Oseretsky Test of Motor Proficiency Short Form (BOT-S) confirmed previous findings in the literature that the older motor impaired children did not perform as well as normally developing peers. A difference in age-related changes in motor performance was found in the clumsy group when compared with the scores of the other motor impaired children. Clumsy younger children's motor performance scores were closer to the other motor impaired children, whereas the older clumsy children obtained much higher motor performance scores than the other motor impaired children (Appendix A, Part 3 gives more details of the results). The similarities and differences for each of these groups of motor impaired children will be discussed in the next section.

Clumsy children

Of particular interest was the finding that clumsy children have a pattern of age-related improvement in performance which is different from the pattern for children who are intellectually disabled or have Down syndrome. For example, younger clumsy children scored significantly lower than their intellectually disabled and Down syndrome peers in the dynamic balance task and only scored significantly higher in catching. Their scores in the agility run were also significantly higher than children with Down syndrome, but not intellectually disabled children. On the other tests they were not significantly different (i.e. in static balance, jumping and clapping hands, and standing broad jump).

In contrast, the older clumsy children's motor performance was significantly better than their age peers in the two other motor impaired groups, on tests measuring agility run, static balance, dynamic balance, jump and clap hands, and standing broad jump. The only item in which there was no significant difference among the motor impaired children was the bilateral coordination task of tapping the feet while making circles with the fingers (as most of the children could not perform this task).

The results for clumsy children appear to indicate that the younger children classified as clumsy showed a different pattern of motor impairment than the older children. The younger clumsy group had particular deficits in balance and bilateral coordination, and strength when compared with the older clumsy group. Additionally, the clumsy children in the younger group did not obtain scores that were significantly higher than age peers who are intellectually disabled or have Down syndrome in nearly every other item on the test, whereas the older clumsy children were superior in all items to the other groups of motor impaired children (Appendix A, Part 3).

Children who are intellectually disabled or have Down syndrome

The pattern of deficit in motor performance for children who are intellectually disabled, with or without Down syndrome, was similar for both the younger and older groups of children which suggests that these children are developmentally delayed, when compared with normally coordinated children. This is because there appears to be a steady improvement from the younger to the older age group. Also of interest is the fact that children with Down syndrome, when compared with similarly intellectually disabled children, obtained comparable motor performance scores in all items measured, with the exception of their significantly lower performance on the agility run. Their slower speed in running and agility may be related to postural problems and gait abnormalities which are common in children with Down syndrome (Lydic and Steele, 1979; Parker and Bronks, 1980; Parker, Bronks and Snyder, 1986).

The finding that, apart from running speed, there is almost no difference in motor performance between the intellectually disabled and Down syndrome groups suggests that the underlying inherent abnormalities of children with Down syndrome affect motor performance less than was previously thought. Additionally, it would appear that these results provide further evidence that physique and stature may not greatly influence motor performance, because children with Down syndrome tend to have an endomorphic body build, yet their motor performance is more similar than dissimilar to other children who have a more normal body build.

Results from this study for the intellectually disabled and Down syndrome groups are also in agreement with those reported by Henderson, Morris and Ray (1981), who found the only significant difference in gross motor performance between the two categories of intellectually disabled children was in the agility and locomotor agility tasks. The data, from the study, however, do not support some of the results found by Connolly and Michael (1986), who measured motor performance of Down syndrome and intellectually disabled boys and girls in middle childhood. These authors found, on the full version of the BOT that intellectually disabled children were significantly better in performance than children with Down syndrome on subtests of running speed and agility, strength, visual motor control, and upper limb speed and dexterity. Nevertheless, the present results support Connolly and Michael's findings, that the tests of bilateral coordination and upper limb coordination did not distinguish between the two groups and that in this study, the intellectually disabled children were only better than the Down syndrome group in the item measuring running speed and agility.

In this study, therefore, as in the other studies of motor performance (using the Bruininks–Oseretsky Test of Motor Performance) the differences between intellectually disabled and Down syndrome groups are not consistent. Part of the discrepancy across studies may be due to the fact that the results of Connolly and Michael's study are based on the full BOT whereas the study reported here only compared performance on five of eight subtests which comprise the Short Form. The present results suggest, however, that when comparing motor performance between similarly intellectually disabled children, with and without Down syndrome, the major difference appears to occur in tasks measuring running speed and agility.

CONCLUSION FROM THE STUDY

1. This study highlights differences in motor performance among children in early and middle childhood, who are clumsy, intellectually disabled or who have Down syndrome.
2. Another important finding from this study is the relatively poor performance of younger clumsy children when compared with older clumsy children. Younger clumsy children's motor performance patterns differed, in comparison with the older clumsy children, in terms of poor balance, bilateral coordination and strength. There was also a discrepancy in improvement on performance of motor tasks, in younger and older clumsy children in comparison with peers who are intellectually disabled or have Down syndrome, in that their improvement is proportionally greater.
3. A comparison of the data for normally developing children suggests that all the motor impaired children, who participated in the study, could also be called developmentally delayed because of their overall lower scores than the normally developing children. The younger clumsy children, for example, obtained a mean total score on the subtests 1–5 of the BOT-S, which was more than 2 standard

deviations lower than the group of normally developing children aged 4 years 7 months. The older clumsy group obtained a mean total score on the five subtests of 27.29, which is slightly lower than the 6 years 7 months old normally developing children's scores.

4. Younger intellectually disabled children obtained a mean total score of 12.83, which is more than two standard deviations below the mean total score for normally developing children aged 4 years 7 months. Their peers with Down syndrome were more than 3 standard deviations below the mean. The older groups of children with intellectual disability and Down syndrome obtained mean total scores which were more than 3 standard deviations below the mean total score for normally developing children aged 6 years 7 months.
5. It must be reiterated, however, that a general finding of developmental delay is partly due to the nature of motor performance tests, because the test used measured movement skills in terms of age-referenced norms. In this study, therefore, it was expected that children with an intellectual disability would obtain lower scores, as they tend to perform skills at a level closer to their mental rather than their chronological age. Nevertheless, the finding of a marked difference in scores between younger and older clumsy children provides some evidence that these children might progress in their motor performance at a rate different from their intellectually disabled, motor impaired peers.

In conclusion, on the basis of the motor performance data it is not possible to determine whether the results confirm a developmental delay or difference hypothesis, even though specific areas have been identified that need attention in adapted motor programmes for similarly impaired children. To gain a clearer picture of the movement behaviour of motor impaired children, other measures such as the fundamental movement pattern check-list need to be used, which examine quality of movement and provide information about children's levels of maturation. Motor control measures are also considered important because they examine advanced control processes which affect both the quality as well as the ability to perform motor tasks (i.e. a quantitative measure). These two measures of movement behaviour are examined in subsequent chapters, in order to develop a more comprehensive picture of motor impaired children's movement behaviour. The next measure of motor development to be examined in this book is that of fundamental movement patterns.

REFERENCES

Barden, H.S. (1985) Dentition and other aspects of growth and development, in *Current Approaches to Down's Syndrome* (eds D. Lane and B. Stratford), Rinehart & Winston, London, pp. 71–84.

Branta, C., Haubenstricker, J. and Seefeldt, V. (1984) Age changes in motor skills during childhood and adolescence. *Exercise and Sport Science Review*, **12**, 467–520.

Broadhead, G.D. and Church, G.E. (1985) Movement characteristics of preschool children. *Research Quarterly for Exercise and Sport*, **56**, 208–14.

Bruininks, R. (1978) *Bruininks–Oseretsky Test of Motor Proficiency: Examiners Manual*. American Guidance Services, Circle Pines, MN.

Bullock, M.I. and Watter, P. (1984) Patterns of motor development in children with minimal cerebral dysfunction, in *Tenth International Congress World Federation for Physical Therapy*, Link Printing, Sydney, pp. 280–4.

Connolly, B.H. and Michael, B.T. (1986) Performance of retarded children with and without Down's syndrome, on the Bruininks–Oseretsky Test of Motor Proficiency. *Physical Therapy*, **66**, 344–8.

Cooke, R.E. (1984) Atlantoaxial instability in individuals with Down's Syndrome. *Adapted Physical Activity Quarterly*, **1**, 194–6.

Cratty, B.J. (1979) *Perceptual and Motor Development in Infants and Young Children*. Prentice-Hall, Englewood Cliffs, NJ.

Cronk, C.E. (1978) Growth in children with Down's Syndrome: birth to age 3 years. *Pediatrics*, **61**, 564–8.

Cronk, C.E., Chumlea, C. and Roche, A.F. (1985) Assessment of overweight children with Trisomy 21. *American Journal of Mental Deficiency*, **89**, 433–6.

De Oreo, K.L. (1974) The performance and development of fundamental motor skills in preschool children, in *Psychology of Motor Behavior and Sport* (eds G.A. Wade and R. Martens), Human Kinetics, Champaign, IL, pp. 327–43.

Dobbins, D.A . and Rarick, G. L. (1976) Separation potential of educable retarded and intellectually normal boys as a function of motor performance *Research Quarterly*, **47**, 346–56.

Donoghue, E.C., Kirkman, B.H., Bullmore, G.H.L. *et al.* (1970) Some factors affecting age of walking in a mentally retarded population. *Developmental Medicine and Child Neurology*, **12**, 781–92.

Dyer, S., Gunn, P., Rauh, H. and Berry, P. (1990) Motor development in Down Syndrome children: an analysis of the motor scale of the Bayley Scales of Infant Development, in *Motor Development in Children: Aspects of Coordination and Control*, (eds M.G. Wade and H.T.A. Whiting), Martinus Nijhoff, Dordrecht, ppp. 107–21.

Eckert, H.M. and Rarick, G.L. (1976) Stabilometer performance of educable mentally retarded and normal children. *Research Quarterly*, **47**, 619–23.

Erbaugh, S.J. (1984) The relationship of stability performance and the physical growth characteristics of preschool children. *Research Quarterly for Exercise and Sport*, **55**, 8–16.

Espenchade, A.S. and Eckert, H.M. (1980) *Motor Development*, Charles E. Merrill, Columbus, OH.

Francis, R.J. and Rarick, G.L. (1959) Motor characteristics of the mentally retarded, *American Journal of Mental Deficiency*, **63**, 792–811.

Gillberg, I.C. (1985) Children with minor neurodevelopmental disorders: neurological and neurodevelopmental problems at age 10. *Developmental Medicine and Child Neurology*, **27**, 3–16.

Gubbay, S. (1975) *The Clumsy Child*. W.B. Saunders, London.

Henderson, S.E. (1985) Motor skill development, in *Current Approaches to Down's Syndrome* (eds D. Lane and B. Stratford), Holt, Rinehart & Winston, London, pp. 187–213.

Henderson, S.E. (1987) The assessment of clumsy children: old and new approaches. *Journal of Child Psychology and Psychiatry*, **28**, 511–29.

Henderson, S.E. and Hall, D. (1982) Concomitants of clumsiness in young school children. *Developmental Medicine and Child Neurology*, **24**, 448–60.

Henderson, S.E., Morris, J. and Ray. S. (1981) Performance of Down Syndrome and other retarded children on the Cratty Gross-Motor Test. *American Journal of Mental Deficiency*, **85**, 416–24.

Hills, A.P. (1991) *Physical Growth and Development in Children and Adolescents*, Queensland University of Technology, Brisbane.

Hoare, D. and Larkin, D. (1991) Kinesthetic abilities of clumsy children. *Developmental Medicine and Child Neurology*, **33**, 671–8.

Keogh, J., Sugden, D., Reynard, C.L. and Calkins, J.A. (1979) Identification of clumsy children: comparisons and comments. *Journal of Human Movement Studies*, **5**, 32–41.

Kerr, R. and Blais, C. (1985) Motor skill acquisition by individuals with Down's Syndrome. *American Journal of Mental Deficiency*, **90**, 313–18.

Kirk, S.A. and Gallagher, J.J. (1986) *Educating Exceptional Children*, Houghton Mifflin, Boston.

Larkin, D. and Hoare, D. (1991) *Out of Step*, The University of Western Australia, Nedlands.

Larkin, D. and Hoare, D. (1992) The movement approach: a window to understanding the clumsy child, in *Approaches to The Study of Motor Control and Learning* (ed. J.J. Summers), North Holland, Elsevier Science, Amsterdam, pp. 413–40.

Le Blanc, D., French, R. and Shultz, B. (1977) Static and dynamic balance skills of trainable children with Down's Syndrome. *Perceptual and Motor Skills*, **45**, 641–2.

Liemohn, W.P. and Knapczyk, D.R. (1974) Factor analysis of gross and fine motor ability in developmentally disabled children. *Research Quarterly*, **45**, 424–32.

Lockwood, R.J. (1987) New methods in the study of the poorly coordinated child. Paper presented at *The International Forum for Programs, and Workshops on Physical Activity for the Disabled*. Brisbane, Australia.

Losse, A., Henderson, S.E., Elliman, D. *et al.* (1991) Clumsiness in children do they grow out of it? A ten year follow-up study. *Developmental Medicine and Child Neurology*, **44**, 55–69.

Lydic, J.S. and Steele, C. (1979) Assessment of the quality of sitting and gait patterns in children with Down's Syndrome. *Physical Therapy*, **59**, 1489–94.

Mahan, K.T., Diamond, E. and Brown, D. (1983) Podiatric profile of the Down's Syndrome individual, *Journal of the American Podiatry Association*, **73**, 173–9.

Malina, R.M. (1974) Motor development: determinants and the need to consider them, in *Psychology of Motor Behavior and Sport* (eds M.G. Wade and R. Martens), Human Kinetics, Champaign, IL, pp. 294–306.

Malina, R.M. (1981) Growth, maturation and human performance, in *Perspectives on the Academic Discipline of Physical Education*, (ed. G.A. Brooks), Human Kinetics, Champaign, IL, pp. 190–210.

Malina, R.M. (1984) Physical growth and maturation, *Motor Development During Childhood and Adolescence* (ed. J.R. Thomas), Burgess, Minneapolis, pp. 2–26.

McIntire, I. and Dutch, T.M. (1964) Mongolism and generalized hypotonia. *American Journal of Mental Deficiency*, **68**, 669–70.

Molnar, G.E. (1978) Analysis of motor disorder in retarded infants and young children. *American Journal of Mental Deficiency*, **83**, 213–22.

Morris, A.F., Vaughan, S.E. and Vaccaro, P. (1982) Measurements of neuromuscular tone and strength in Down's Syndrome children. *Journal of Mental Deficiency Research*, **26**, 41–6.

Morris, A.M., Williams, J.M., Atwater, A.E. and Wilmore, J.H. (1982) Age and sex differences in motor performance of 3 through 6 year old children. *Research Quarterly for Exercise and Sport*, **53**, 214–21.

Newell, K.M. (1984) Physical constraints to development of motor skills, in *Motor Development During Childhood and Adolescence* (ed. J.R. Thomas), Burgess, Minneapolis, pp. 105–20.

O'Brien, C.C. (1988) Motor development in clumsy, intellectually disabled and Down's Syndrome children: a comparative study. Unpublished PhD thesis, University of Queensland.

O'Brien, C.C. and Hayes, A. (1989) Motor development in early childhood of clumsy, intellectually disabled and Down's Syndrome children. *The ACHPER National Journal* **124**, 15–19.

Paine, R.S. (1962) Minimal chronic brain syndrome in children. *Developmental Medicine and Child Neurology*, **4**, 21–7.

Parker, A.W. and Bronks, R. (1980) Gait of children with Down's Syndrome. *Archives of Physical Medicine and Rehabilitation*, **61**, 345–51.

Parker, A.W., Bronks, R. and Snyder, C.W. (1986) Walking patterns in Down's Syndrome. *Journal of Mental Deficiency Research*, **30**, 317–30.

Parker, A.W. and James, B. (1985) Age changes in the flexibility of Down's Syndrome children. *Journal of Mental Deficiency Research*, **29**, 207–18.

Paine, R.S., Werry, J.S. and Quay, H.C. (1968) A study of minimal cerebral dysfunction. *Developmental Medicine and Child Neurology*, **10**, 21–7.

Rarick, G.L. (1981) The emergence of the study of human motor development, in *Perspectives on the Academic Discipline of Physical Education*, (ed. G.A. Brooks), Human Kinetics, Champaign, IL, pp. 163–89.

Rarick, G.L. (1982) Descriptive research and process-oriented explanations of the motor development of children, in *The Development of Movement Control and Co-ordination*, (eds J.A.S. Kelso and J.E. Clark), John Wiley, Chichester.

Rarick, G.L., Dobbins, D.A. and Broadhead, G.D. (1976) *The Motor Domain and its Correlates in Educationally Handicapped Children*, Prentice Hall, Englewood Cliffs, NJ.

Semine, A.A., Ertel, A.N., Goldberg, M.J. and Bull, M.J. (1978) Cervical-spine instability in children with Down Syndrome (Trisomy 21). *Journal of Bone and Joint Surgery*, **60-A**, 649–52.

Share, J. and French, R. (1982) *Motor Development of Down's Syndrome Children: Birth to 6 Years*. US Department of Education, National Institute of Education Research.

Sherrill, C. (1986) *Adapted Physical Education and Recreation*, Wm. C. Brown, Iowa.

Smoll, F.L. (1982) Developmental kinesiology: towards a subdiscipline focusing on motor development, in *The Development of Movement Control and Coordination*, (eds J.A.S. Kelso and J.E. Clark), John Wiley, New York, pp. 319–27.

Stott, D.H., Henderson, S.E. and Moyes, F.A. (1986) The Henderson Revision of the Test of Motor Impairment – a comprehensive approach to assessment. *Adapted Physical Activity Quarterly*, **3**, 204–16.

Winnick, J.P. and Short, F.X. (1991) A comparison of the physical fitness of nonretarded and mildly mentally retarded adolescents with cerebral palsy. *Adapted Physical Activity Quarterly*, **8**, 43–56.

Woollacott, M.H. (1993) Normal and abnormal development of posture control in children. Paper presented at *The 9th International Symposium on Adapted Physical Activity*, Yokohama, Japan, August, 1993.

4

Fundamental movement patterns

This chapter traces changes in the fundamental intratask movement patterns (as defined in Chapter 1) of walking, running jumping, catching and throwing, in normally developing children. The basic levels of the movement patterns are characteristic of early childhood (4–7 years) and the mature patterns generally occur in middle childhood (8–12 years). Fundamental movement patterns provide a qualitative measure of children's motor development. These measures extend our knowledge of children's movement behaviour by providing information about how certain children are performing, even though they may be performing at a level below their age norm.

The fundamental movement patterns that are presented in this book were developed over a two-year period (O'Brien and Hayes, 1989). Fundamental movement patterns are considered important from developmental, biomechanical, motor learning and control perspectives. Movement pattern check-lists provide an appropriate instrument for observing children's walking, running, jumping, catching and throwing patterns in naturalistic and more formal settings (Chapter 5). The literature used in developing these instruments is presented in this chapter. Before each of the areas dealing with a specific movement pattern is reviewed, there is a brief general overview of motor development and fundamental movement patterns.

OVERVIEW

Developmental changes should satisfy three requirements;

they should be orderly, directional and stable (Fischer and Lazerson, 1984). Of the many changes which occur with time, only those which satisfy the following criteria are considered developmental: (a) they have some sequential order, (b) they are based on components from a preceding level in the sequence and (c) they have features which are intransient (Fischer and Lazerson, 1984).

Early researchers charted the developmental progression in movement sequences such as walking, running (Gesell, 1973; McGraw, 1966; Sinclair, 1973) and throwing (Wellman, 1937; Wild, 1938). They researched large numbers of children, using detailed observations, which have not been repeated. They noted that a number of movements in young children evolve in a similar manner in nearly all children. For this reason such sequences are usually called fundamental movement patterns. Changes in fundamental movement patterns were considered by these early researchers to occur in an abrupt manner. The theoretical concept to describe these changes was known throughout the developmental literature as stages of development, and has also been applied to changes in other areas of development, such as cognitive development.

In line with modern theories those changes in motor development resulting in a different configuration of the fundamental movement pattern are called different levels of development. The shift in terminology is due to a different conceptual approach in developmental theory. When this approach is applied to motor development, levels of development encompass the theoretical position that within a total movement sequence, the number of components that make up that sequence may progress to a more complex form at different rates. In the throwing pattern for example, some children at the same overall level (e.g., level 3), may have a less mature trunk and arm action and others may have a less mature leg action, but overall their total action is closer to level 3.

Fundamental movement patterns are defined as having movements that involve one or more joints. They have similar configurations in the order and timing of the components, that make up recognized patterns such as walking, running, jumping, catching and throwing (Rarick, 1982). Such patterns can range from relatively simple movements, that occur in the early arm movements in underarm throwing, to the highly complex organization of movement in the mature running pattern. Although movement patterns may appear similar, there are differences between people in terms of kinematic variables (i.e., horizontal, vertical and rotational displacements, velocities and acceleration), and in terms of the kinetic variables (i.e., work, power and potential energy) (Wickstrom, 1983; Winter, 1983).

Movement patterns have often been divided into a hierarchical order from the most basic to the most complex configurations of the movement (Roberton, 1977a, b, 1984; Seefeldt, 1979; Sinclair, 1973; Wickstrom, 1977, 1983; Wild, 1938). This progression of fundamental movement patterns was once considered to occur in a series of abrupt changes which were labelled stages of development. It is considered by the authors, however, that current motor developmentalists should move away from the concept of stages to the more flexible notion of levels of proficiency between, and within, a movement pattern. That is, movement pattern may progress from a simple to a more complex form with development, and involve considerable scope for individual differences. In the throwing pattern, for example, a group of children may be classified as being at the second level of development in their overall pattern, but some may have a less mature arm action and others a less mature leg action than their peers.

Basic or fundamental movement patterns are the first movements from which skilled movements are derived. Early researchers regarded the first five years of life as the period in which most children normally acquire and refine fundamental movement patterns (Wickstrom, 1983). Current knowledge suggests that more mature levels of these patterns do not emerge until approximately 7 years of age (Clark and Whitall, 1989; Halverson and Williams, 1985; Roberton 1978, 1984; Seefeldt and Haubenstricker, 1982).

Where appropriate, the approximate age of the attainment by normally developing children, for each of the various movement levels will be given throughout the chapter. It must be remembered, though, that these patterns are developmental and that the mature form represents a level of skill that is not only dependent on maturation and biological processes, but also on a range of environmental and experiential factors, in particular the extent of practice. This suggests, that although mature levels in a movement sequence represent the most complex form of a particular pattern, these levels are generally achieved during middle childhood. Nevertheless, the mature form may never be attained by some people because of insufficient practice or physical, neurological or cognitive limitations (Wickstrom, 1983).

In this book developmental levels were derived from a review of literature on the fundamental movement patterns of walking, running, jumping, catching and throwing. Once the developmental progressions were derived they were tested on normally developing children (Halverson and Roberton, 1978; O'Brien, 1988). This procedure was considered essential because it verified preliminary sequences, that were developed by the authors and were then used to identify developmental delays or developmental differences in exceptional children.

The following section reviews the literature on the normal development of each of the fundamental movement patterns for walking, running, jumping, catching and throwing.

WALKING

Walking, or bipedal locomotion in humans, is achieved by alternate movements of the lower limbs, with one foot in continuous contact with the ground (Wickstrom, 1977). Achievement of walking is an extremely important milestone because it indicates that infants are developing control over their postural stability and their interlimb coordination. Infants find that walking is a very difficult movement skill, since it requires control over an unstable body, which is supported for approximately 80% of total stance time by only one of the lower limbs (Winter, 1983). Because walking is such a universal, but difficult skill, the study of its progression is especially important not only from a developmental perspective, but also to obtain an understanding of movement development in motor impaired children (Wheelwright *et al.*, 1993).

Prewalking stages were outlined by Shirley (1931) and McGraw (1966). From these and subsequent studies it is evident that attainment of the least mature phase of erect locomotion is innate in origin, and is dependent upon development of the balance mechanisms, interlimb control, visual input, and sufficient strength of the extensor muscles in the lower limbs and back (Thelen, Ulrich and Jensen, 1989; Bril and Breneire, 1992). Generally, children who are advanced in the developmental milestones that demonstrate control over gravity, such as sitting and crawling, will walk before children of the same chronological age who are less advanced (Burnett and Johnson, 1971a). Other physiological factors such as the physique of the child and the amount of fat tissue will influence the age of onset of walking (Cratty, 1979).

Precarious balance causes infants to appear unsteady and fall easily when they first walk. To compensate for poor dynamic balance the infant usually walks with the legs wide apart (to achieve a wide base of support) and holds the arms in a fixed sideways position, generally above shoulder height. At this level of development children have a rigid body and a jerky and irregular stepping action, with marked flexion at the knees and hips (though some children have hip flexion and relatively little flexion in the knees). They have a heavy, flat foot contact with the ground and marked sideways sway with each step as they try to maintain a balanced position (Bril and Breneire, 1992; Clark and Whitall, 1989; McGraw, 1966; Wickstrom, 1977).

Research studies related to developmental changes in the walking pattern

Recent research has shown that early walking can be divided into two distinct phases during children's first two years of walking (Bril and Breneire, 1992). The first phase, which lasts for 3–6 months, is characterized by great variability in all the gait parameters but especially the width the legs are apart and the length of the step. It is also possible that children use the wide stride width to produce the disequilibrium needed for a single support phase (Bril and Breneire, 1992, p. 113). The second phase, which lasts for about 18 months, is distinguished by greater stability (tuning) of gait parameters and a narrowing of the width of the base of support.

According to other researchers, once the walking pattern has appeared the width of the base of support decreases rapidly and there is an increase in stride length. In addition, pelvic rotation, knee flexion at mid stance, the foot and knee mechanism and lateral displacement of the pelvis all contributed to control of postural stability. All these elements of the gait pattern had appeared by about 29 months of age (Burnett and Johnson, 1971, a,b).

In another cross-sectional study, a biomechanical analysis was conducted on the characteristics of the walking pattern in children aged between 1 and 7 years. Investigators examined angular rotations of the limb segments, and step length, cadence, walking velocity and duration of single leg stance (Sutherland *et al.*, 1980). They found that the five important determinants of a mature gait are duration of single-leg stance, walking velocity, cadence, step length and the ratio of pelvic spread to ankle spread. Their data also confirmed that heel strike, knee flexion and reciprocal arm swing are present in children by 3 years of age.

Maturational and growth factors appear to influence other aspects of the walking pattern. These include step length, walking velocity and single limb support and cadence (number of steps per unit of time). These later-developing aspects of gait, according to Sutherland *et al.* (1980), are better indicators of mature gait than the joint angle patterns, even though they are more difficult to observe than changes in heel-strike and upper and lower limb actions. Some of these characteristics of the movement pattern of walking which have been identified will be discussed in the next section.

Characteristics of the walking pattern

Stance on a single limb reflects the ability to maintain stability of the body. The duration of single limb stance decreases rapidly from onset of walking until 2 years 6 months of age, when the step rate is constant. Rate of increase in walking speed levels out after 3 years 6 months and cadence decreases with age (Sutherland *et al.*, 1980). A higher cadence, shorter stride length, leg swing and single support duration has been found in 5 year olds in comparison with 6 and 7 year olds, according to Brown and Parker (1992). These authors did not find any significant difference among 5, 6 and 7 year olds in free walking velocity, stride length, ratio of step length to length of the lower limb, on time spent on one limb, on both limbs and the differences in the timing between each leg step (Brown and Parker, 1992).

The average step length in children increases from 10 to 11.5 inches between 1 and 2 years of age and from 13 to 15 inches between three and four years of age (Sutherland *et al.*, 1980). In fact it has been reported that between 11 months and 14 years, average step length was maintained at 38% of the child's height (Wickstrom 1983) and in another study it was 43% of the child's height (Wheelwright *et al.*, 1993). Together with an increase in stride length, there are changes in foot placement from flat foot contact with the ground to out-toeing, to a relatively straight foot placement (Espenchade and Eckert, 1980) and an increased angle at the ankle as body support was transfered to the forward limb (dorsiflexion) (Brown and Parker, 1992). In-toeing has also been reported as relatively common (Wickstrom, 1983). The base of support changes from being wider than the body and the average step length, at onset of walking to being within the limits of the body and remaining at that width from about 3 years of age (Bril and Breneire, 1992; Sutherland *et al.*, 1980).

There are developmental changes, until 2 years of age, in the flexion (movement of the limb in towards the body), and extension (straightening of the limb) at the hip, in terms of a decrease in flexion and a rapid increase in the extension angle. Children of 5 years, have greater hip adduction in the single support phase, in comparison with 7 year olds who have greater hip abduction (Brown and Parker, 1992). There is then a steady change in hip angle until about 7 years of age when the hip flexion and extension pattern is similar to that of an adult. Pelvic tilt also decreases rapidly from early onset of walking until about 2 years of age when the pelvic tilt angle is the same as that of the mature pattern (Wickstrom, 1983).

Other changes in the appearance of the walking pattern are largely due to progressive changes in the action at the knee and ankle joints. At first the knee, both in the support and swing phase, is slightly flexed, and there is little extension in the ankle movement. Once heel-toe contact appears this is followed by knee-lock (or extension of the knee) of the support leg. This progression leads to the next phase, where there is increased ankle extension, knee flexion at mid-stance and full knee extension before the push-off phase of the supporting leg. These flexion and extension changes in the hip, knee and ankle mechanism are responsible for the smooth transfer of weight which is characteristic of the mature walking pattern (Burnett and Johnson, 1971b; Clark and Whitall, 1989).

Trunk inclination decreases as balance improves and the arm action changes from a 'high guard position' at onset of walking, to arms held by the side with little swing. Further progression is from arm swing at the forearm to a contralateral arm action, which is initiated from the shoulder, in the mature pattern (McClenaghan and Gallahue, 1978; McGraw, 1966; Wickstrom, 1977, 1983).

It would appear that gait asymmetry of 8–10% is part of the normal pattern. Variability in gait parameters among normally developing children aged from 3 to 18 years of age, has been reported as 1% for leg swing time and average foot-width and step length between the left and right limbs, whereas a 9% decrease in double support time has been reported following the left stride in comparison with the right stride (Wheelwright *et al.*, 1993).

The findings of the literature review on walking patterns have been collated in Chapter 5 and presented pictorially as sequences, which can be used as criteria for observational assessments. For observational purposes it is convenient to divide the progression into various levels or developmental components, from the most basic to the most mature patterns of walking. It must be remembered, though, that children's walking patterns change gradually, rather than abruptly, from one level to the next.

Summary of changes in the walking pattern

Following the immature phase (at approximately 2 years of age), there is less muscle tension evident, partly because of improved balance control and relaxation of co-contraction of the muscles. The pattern appears less jerky than at the previous developmental level and there is greater consistency of stride action, both in the action of each leg and the length of stride. The forward leg 'locks' at the knee after the heel first contacts the ground. The base of support of the body is about the same width as the trunk, out-toeing of the feet decreases and the arms are held by the side with some armswing (Clark and

Whitall, 1989; O'Brien, 1991; Sutherland *et al.*, 1980; Thelen, Ulrich and Jensen, 1989; Wickstrom, 1977).

By 4–5 years of age all elements of the mature pattern are present. Consistency in leg action and stride length is evident. There is smooth transfer of weight because of well-developed hip-knee-ankle mechanisms. When the forward leg makes contact with the ground, the knee is slightly flexed, followed by extension of the knee during the support phase. The centre of gravity of the body remains relatively constant so that there is far less vertical displacement than at the previous levels. Only a small amount of pelvic rotation is present to facilitate transfer of weight. The arm swing is in opposition to the forward leg (contralateral action), though one arm is usually swung more than the other (Thelen, Ulrich and Jensen, 1989; Wickstrom, 1977).

The mature walking pattern, which is usually present in children at about 7 years of age, is characterized by a smooth, rhythmical action at the ankle, knee and hip joints. There is a consistent stride length, a decrease in cadence in comparison with earlier levels of the walking pattern and the arms move in opposition to the legs to counteract lateral rotation of the body (Brown and Parker, 1992; O'Brien, 1988; Sutherland *et al.*, 1980; Wickstrom, 1983).

Figure 5.1 a–d (pp.114–17) is a pictorial representation of the development of walking in normally developing children.

RUNNING

Running is a fundamental locomotor pattern which is similar to walking in terms of the limb pattern and in the transfer of weight from one foot to the other. Running generally is not achieved by children before 18 months of age because of insufficient strength and an inability to maintain balance (Wickstrom, 1983). When running does appear it is in a less mature form than the locomotor pattern of walking concurrently exhibited by the same child (Burnett and Johnson, 1971a; Clark and Whitall, 1989). The distinctive characteristic of running is that there is a period during the leg cycle when there is no foot in contact with the ground (non-support phase). Running is actually a series of jumps with the body weight supported on one foot, followed by an airborne phase, then the body weight is supported on the opposite foot (Wickstrom, 1977, 1983).

Strength, postural control and interlimb coordination must be developed sufficiently in the infant, so that the limbs are able to be coordinated at the increased speed necessary for running. Running also requires greater strength in the legs, so that the body can be propelled forward and become airborne at the same time. In addition, balance mechanisms must be developed to a point where the infant can maintain balance during the non-support phase of the cycle and then transfer weight smoothly to the forward leg (Espenchade and Eckert, 1980).

In the most basic running pattern, the body is upright, arms hang down by the side and, if there is any armswing, it is with a fairly straight arm and is mainly used to help maintain balance (McClenaghan and Gallahue, 1978). This type of pattern is achieved in most children by about 18 months to two years of age (Gesell, 1973). As running speed increases, the stride is lengthened and the airborne phase is extended. Some of the changes which occur are that the leg is brought forward faster and with a greater angle at the knee joint, the heel begins to contact the ground first, there is also a faster extension pattern in the back leg and a stronger push-off. The arms are swung with increased vigour, both backwards and forwards, the swing is initiated from the shoulder rather than at the elbow, and the action is characterized by a bent elbow (Wickstrom, 1983).

Research studies related to developmental changes in the running pattern

Wickstrom (1983) in summarizing a series of unpublished doctoral and masters dissertations, reported the following age-related trends in running (p. 47). There is:

1. an increase in the length of running stride;
2. a decrease in the relative amount of vertical movement in each stride;
3. an increase in hip, knee and ankle extension at take-off;
4. an increase in the proportion of time in the non-support phase of the stride;

5. an increase in the closeness of the heel to the buttock on the forward swing;
6. an increase in the height of the forward knee at take-off;
7. a decrease in the relative distance that the support foot is ahead of the centre of gravity of the body at contact.

Another study of the running patterns of 2, 4 and 6 year old children found that the 2 year olds had only just achieved a running pattern (i.e., they had achieved an elementary air-borne phase), 4 year olds had all the basic elements and 6 year olds had movement patterns which had all the elements of the mature running pattern (Fortney, 1983). Wickstrom also found that step length increased with age. Despite these reported differences, in levels of maturity of running in the 4 and 6 year old groups, they had similar running speed. Both the 4 and 6 year old groups, however, were faster than the 2 year old group. In addition, in each group the movement patterns of the girls did not differ significantly from those of the boys. Fortney (1983), nevertheless, found that there were major differences in the running pattern, in terms of the action of the leg swinging forward at the knee and ankle joint, between the 2 and 6 year olds groups. The data suggest that developmental changes in the running pattern, between 2 and 4 years of age, are related to an increase in knee flexion and increased ankle plantar flexion in the swinging leg. There also appear to be gender differences, as boys had a greater range of motion and greater flexion in the swinging hip in comparison with the girls' running action.

The results of Fortney's (1983) study are interesting because, even though there was no significant difference in speed between girls and boys, there was a significant difference in hip action between boys and girls up to 6 years of age. He argued that this difference in the hip action might offer some clue as to why boys have a faster running speed than girls in middle childhood. Particularly, as it has been shown that more mature runners, and elite athletes, have greater flexion in the knee of the swinging leg and a larger angle at push-off, and the leg is swung forward in a higher position than less skilful runners (McClenaghan and Gallahue, 1978).

Summary of changes in the running pattern

Once the basic running pattern is present it is subject to numerous changes, as children develop better dynamic balance. For example, the base of support becomes narrower, there is a longer airborne phase and the arms are dropped down to hang at the side of the body (Sinclair, 1973). In terms of limb control there is a more fluent leg action and during the push-off phase there is an increased application of force. Wickstrom (1983) reported that, at this level of running (approx. age 2–3 years), there is often asymmetry in the leg action with a longer airborne phase and a greater stride length of one leg than the other. There is little or no voluntary arm-swing, except a small amount of movement at the elbow joints. Elements of heel–toe contact or, less often, ball of the foot contact may be present. Stride length has also increased, but there is still some evidence of immature motor control, as children of approximately 3–4 years of age have difficulty in stopping, starting and turning (Wickstrom, 1977, 1983).

At the next level, elements such as the ankle, knee and hip action and the timing of various subroutines are closer to the mature level than the basic pattern (Espenchade and Eckert, 1980; Fortney, 1983). Some components which are not present in the mature pattern are evident, such as marked pelvic rotation with each stride and the tendency to hook the forward swinging arm in towards the middle of the body and out away from the body on the backswing (Wickstrom, 1983).

In the mature running pattern, the support foot contacts the ground directly under the body, while initial contact with the ground in fast sprinting is with the heel or ball of the foot. Knee flexion follows ground contact, which maximizes horizontal progression and the arm is swung from the shoulder, with a bent elbow. The mature running pattern is characterized by increased hip extension at take-off and greater knee flexion in the forward swing. There is the appearance of greater body lean because of greater stride length and angle, at push-off, of the back leg (Wickstrom, 1977, 1983).

A pictorial developmental profile, which summarizes this material on the running patterns is found in Figure 5.2 a–d (pp. 120–3).

JUMPING

A jump is characterized by the ability to extend one or both legs with enough force to catapult the body into the air. Jumping is a more complex locomotor skill than running, mainly because the body is airborne for a longer time. This fact alone places greater demands on maturity of the underlying balance, proprioceptive and kinaesthetic feedback mechanisms (Hellebrandt *et al.*, 1961). Furthermore, the limb movements in all but the basic patterns are markedly different from the running and walking patterns. In jumping, both upper limbs and lower limbs move in synchrony (mainly on a vertical axis), to counteract the effects of instability of the body. Additionally, the body is maintained in a balanced position for extended periods, both in the air, in preparation for landing and during the actual landing.

The precursor of the jumping pattern is characterized by a one foot step down from a height, with little or no airborne phase. According to Espenchade and Eckert (1980), the child modifies the walking pattern for his first attempts at jumping. This means that in the basic pattern the child is merely stepping down from something and the arms are used only for balance. Subsequent changes which occur to this level of jumping are related to improved balance and interlimb control. This is shown behaviourally by the child being able to propel the body into the air from a two foot take-off in the standing broadjump and to execute a two foot landing. The arms and legs are used bilaterally in this action. The arms are also used in the take-off action, they counteract vertical instability in the air and are used to stabilize the body on landing (Wickstrom, 1977).

Research studies related to developmental changes in the jumping pattern

Wickstrom (1983) has identified a number of developmental changes in the standing broadjump (pp. 78–9). These are:

1. an increase in the preliminary crouch;
2. an increase in the forward swing in the arms at the anteroposterior plane;

3. a decrease in take-off angle;
4. an increase in total body extension at take-off;
5. an increase in thigh flexion during flight;
6. a decrease in the angle of the leg at the instant of landing.

Early jumping patterns are usually demonstrated by children at about 17 months of age, whereas a two foot take-off for the standing broad jump is generally achieved by 21 months of age. This information was obtained from a study which analysed jumping patterns using filmed data of 14 boys from age 6 years to age 10–11 years (Hellebrandt *et al.*, 1961). These authors also claimed that because the leg action at this basic level was so stereotyped, it indicated that these early jumping patterns are innate in origin. They also argued that changes in the head position, during the jump, were very important because the authors considered that early movements of the head and arms are a result of the continuing influence of the tonic neck reflex upon upper limb movement patterns. This type of action is demonstrated, in their opinion, in immature jumping patterns when the head is extended, and as a consequence there is a backward and 'winging' action of the arms (Hellebrandt *et al.*, 1961).

Developmental differences in the take-off parameters, and body configuration at take-off, in the standing long jump have also been investigated in children aged 3, 4, 5, 6 and 7 years by Phillips, Clark and Petersen (1985). Their findings were that at take-off there were no significant age-related differences in ankle, knee and hip joint angles from 3 years to 7 years of age. In contrast, flexion at the shoulder joint increased significantly with age, and there was a tendency for the centre of gravity of the body to be horizontally further away from the toes at take-off. The majority of the significant differences were found between the three year old group and the other groups (Phillips, Clark and Peterson 1985). This suggests that the other groups of children (4, 5, 6 and 7 year olds) had very similar body configurations at take-off, although the older children jumped a greater distance than the younger ones. The level of performance increased from the younger to the older children.

Another study examined differences in components of the standing broad jump between skilled (elite) and non-skilled women athletes (Zimmerman, 1956). Major differences were found in the ankle, knee and hip action. Skilled jumpers had significantly greater hip and ankle flexion, and knee and ankle extension, than the unskilled group. Also, skilled jumpers did not have as great an angle, at take-off and landing, as the unskilled jumpers. These findings are important because they suggest that even within a mature movement pattern, differences can be found between skilled and less skilled people.

Summary of changes in the jumping pattern

Progression from the precursor to the basic jumping pattern is marked by the child coordinating a two foot take-off, a very brief airborne phase and an unpredictable or asymmetrical two foot landing (Espenchade and Eckert, 1980), with little arm movement. Between 3 and 5 years the normal child assumes a crouch position with inclination of the trunk. The body is then projected high into the air, particularly if the child is jumping off from a height (i.e., there is a large vertical component). The legs are bent at an angle of about 45° during the flight phase of the jump. Then the legs are swung forward, still bent in preparation for the landing. In many children there is a distinctive 'winging' action of the arms, so that the arms after take-off are swung backwards and sideways to resemble 'birdwings'. The head may be extended backwards during flight, but apart from this action there is little head movement during flight (Hellebrandt *et al.*, 1961).

The next level is characterized by a greater horizontal than vertical component in the jump, together with an increased lean forward of the trunk in the take-off and flight phase (Phillips, Clark and Petersen, 1985). The arms are swung forward, above the head and backward on landing and the head is moved forward then backward during the jumping action. Most children take-off in a well-coordinated two-foot action and achieve a balanced landing on both feet. In fact it has been reported that elements of the mature standing broad jump are present sometime between the ages of 6 to 7 years (Phillips, Clark and Petersen, 1985).

The mature standing broad jump is characterized by complete synchronization of the arms, legs and head. There is a deep crouch before take-off, with marked trunk inclination, followed by full body extension and then flexion of the hips and knees during the long airborne phase. The legs are extended and the arms, head and trunk move forward in preparation for the landing. On landing, the knees and hip flex while the trunk and head are dropped forward in an attempt to maintain balance (Wickstrom, 1977, 1983; Zimmerman, 1956).

Pictorial representations of the development of levels of jumping are presented in Figure 5.3 a–d (pp. 126–9).

CATCHING

Catching is defined as the action of the hands and upper body to stop an object that is travelling through the air (Wickstrom, 1983). It is a fundamental gross motor manipulation skill. In comparison with the locomotor patterns, catching forces the person to rely more heavily on external environmental information.

Although children can reach for, and voluntarily grasp, objects towards the end of the first year (Halverson, 1931; O'Brien and Ziviani, 1991), they usually cannot catch a large moving object tossed into the air until they are two and a half to three years of age (Espenchade and Eckert, 1980). Young children have a very variable catching action that varies considerably with the size of the ball and the speed it travels towards them. Generally, children are able to catch a large, light ball more easily than a smaller ball and they cope with slower balls better than fast ones (Espenchade and Eckert, 1980; Sinclair, 1973). A ball tossed into the air is influenced by gravity which makes it harder for a child to catch than one which is rolled or bounced (Espenchade and Eckert, 1980).

The precursor of the catching pattern occurs when the child is able to judge the trajectory of the ball proficiently enough to trap it against part of the body (Espenchade and Eckert, 1980). The toddler from 2 years 6 months to 3 years generally makes no response to a thrown ball unless the toddler is shown how to hold the arms. At this developmental level the child stands facing the thrower with arms extended at waist level, with the palms upwards. If the throw is accurate and lands somewhere on the child's arms, the ball will be scooped in and trapped against the child's body. If the throw does not touch the child's arms, no response will be made to the ball (Sinclair, 1973; McClenaghan and Gallahue, 1978).

Limitations are evident in children's performance on tasks such as catching, which require processing of complex visual, spatial and kinaesthetic information. Some of these limitations will be outlined below.

Research studies related to developmental changes in the catching pattern

Catching is a hand-eye coordination and visual-tracking task that involves complex information processing strategies to enable the person to distinguish the movements of their own body and the movements of the object to be caught (Zanone, 1990). At present there are some data available on how people coordinate eye-to-limb and eye-to-hand coordination in order to catch a moving object. There is evidence, for example, which indicates that adults rely more heavily on proprioceptive information than visual information for control of limb position, before and during the catch. In regard to visual-tracking it has been demonstrated that children, by 5 years of age, can track a slow moving target nearly as well as adults. However, it is not until about 9 years of age that children attain adult levels in judgement of the temporal and spatial characteristics of high-speed tracking (Zanone, 1990).

Although improved tracking of the ball appears to improve catching skills in young children, skilful catchers make judgements about the flight of the ball after a very brief period, so they do not need to track the ball continuously (Whitling, 1969; Strohmeyer, Williams and Schaub-George, 1991). In this regard, an unpublished study is pertinent (by Williams, 1965, reported by Cratty, 1979). The study investigated whether children aged from 5 to 12 years of age could judge the trajectory of a ball after seeing only its initial movement. It was found that 6, 7 and 8 year olds were very inaccurate in their judgements, and it was not until about 9 years of age that the children could accurately judge where the ball was likely to land. A difference between skilled and unskilled adult catchers and the amount of time they need to see the ball has also been reported. Skilful performers only need to sight the ball for approximately 100ms to judge its speed and trajectory accurately (Whiting, Savelsbergh and Faber, 1988).

In regard to the role of vision in orienting the body and hands to intercept the ball, a research finding is that children under 12 years of age need to use peripheral vision more than older children and adults to monitor the correct position of their arms and hands for catching (Davis, 1988). Another study has shown that peripheral vision of the hands, at least 200 ms before the ball is caught, increases interception accuracy. Moreover, this study demonstrated that peripheral vision not only helps accuracy of limb positioning, but also improves the timing of flexion of the fingers around the ball (Smyth and Marriott, 1982). Additional experimental evidence has demonstrated that in children, it is inaccurate positioning of the hands and the grasp of the ball, rather than timing errors in judging the flight of the ball, that cause the most errors in catching (Smyth and Marriott, 1982).

Developmental changes which occur in the catching pattern, like many of the previous patterns have not been verified by longitudinal studies (Wickstrom, 1983). Earlier researchers (e.g., Wellman, 1937) outlined developmental progression on the basis of cross-sectional observational data. Wellman (1937) proposed three levels in the development of catching. The first level was similar to the basic catching pattern outlined in the previous section. The second level was achieved by about 4 years of age, when the ball is caught in the palms of the hand in a sideways clapping action. At the more mature level the arms are used less and the ball is caught with a cupped hand (Espenchade and Eckert, 1980; McClenaghan and Gallahue, 1978). In the mature pattern the hands are moved forward in anticipation of the ball's trajectory. The fingers are angled forward, allowing far more effective closure and control of the ball (Wickstrom, 1983).

Wickstrom (1983) has reported evidence that boys in grades 2 (7 years), 4 (9 years) and 6 (11 years) have more mature catching patterns than girls. He also found that increased ball velocity caused deterioration in the catching performance in children in 2nd and 4th grades, but not in 6th grade. In addition, catching performance was less adversely affected when children had to move laterally to intercept the ball than when they had to move backwards or forwards.

Summary of changes in the catching pattern

Developmental progression from the basic catching pattern, occurs when there is an initial response to the ball. The hands are held out straight and sideways ready to clap the ball between the hands. Another characteristic at this developmental level is to shut the eyes before the ball reaches the hands. Sometimes the head also is turned away from the flight of the ball. On catching the ball, the hands move upwards towards the face and the feet remain in a stationary position, although usually the knees bend as the ball is caught (O'Brien, 1988; Roberton, 1984; Sinclair, 1973).

Children's ability to anticipate the flight of the ball is seen in the next developmental level. The arms are held out in front of the body with elbows bent, hands cupped and fingers extended in preparation to catch the ball. The child is able to move sideways and reach up above the head or below waist height to catch a ball. On catching the ball, the arms are drawn in closer to the body, knees are bent, trunk inclined and a semi-squat position is usually adopted (O'Brien, 1988; Roberton, 1984; Wickstrom, 1983).

In the mature level the person moves with outstretched hands to a position either forward, backward or sideways where he or she will intercept the trajectory of the ball. As the ball is caught there is a backwards or sidewards movement of the arms and shoulders in line with the flight of the ball. Balls thrown at speed can be caught easily and lower limbs adjust completely to the position the body needs to adopt for the ball to be caught (Morris *et al.*, 1982; O'Brien, 1991; Roberton, 1984; Wickstrom, 1983).

Pictorial representations of the developmental sequence of the catching pattern is presented in Figure 5.4 (a–d) (pp. 132–5).

THROWING

Throwing is a gross motor manipulative skill that involves projecting an object into space by using one or two arms (McClenaghan and Gallahue, 1978; Wickstrom, 1977, 1983). Overhand throwing has been validated more extensively than the movement patterns of walking, running, jumping and catching that have already been described. Young infants are first able to release objects at about 10 months of age (Halverson, 1931; O'Brien and Ziviani, 1991). This level of development of the pattern is indicative that the infant has acquired voluntary control of extension of the fingers, over the more dominant grasp pattern.

The initial overhand throwing pattern is only an extension of early release of objects. The child faces the target, with the feet together, lifts the arm at the elbow so that the forearm is at a right angle to the upper arm, from this position the arm is straightened and the ball is released. There is no movement of the lower limbs. The only movement is of the upper limbs and trunk forward and backwards (anterior–posterior plane) (Wild, 1938). Because of its universal appearance the early throwing pattern is considered to be an innate, or inbuilt movement pattern (Halverson, 1931; Wild, 1938).

Characteristic developmental changes which occur in the overhead throwing pattern are increased horizontal trunk rotation, then a unilateral stepping action, followed by opposition in the stepping pattern and marked horizontal trunk rotation (Cratty, 1979; Roberton, 1984; Wild, 1938; Wickstrom, 1983).

Research studies related to developmental changes in the throwing pattern

Two eminent researchers into changes in throwing patterns have been Wild (1938) and Roberton (1977a,b, 1978; Halverson, Roberton and Langendorfer, 1982). Wild (1938) conducted a cross-sectional study of the throwing pattern (using filmed data) on 32 children aged between 2 and 12 years. Velocity measures were taken and verbal descriptions were made of the throw. From the data, Wild formed the opinion that there were certain typical age-related patterns for movements of the arm, legs and whole body. She classified the many patterns into four distinct stages which were as follows:

Stage I. Movements of the body and the arm are almost entirely in the anterio-posterior plane, the body faces the target throughout and the feet remain stationary.
Stage II. Characterized by body and arm movement in a horizontal plane. The arm is held high and oblique over the shoulder, feet remaining stationary during the throw.

Stage III. Throw now has anterio-posterior and horizontal body body movements and the foot is stepped forward in a unilateral pattern with the throwing arm.
Stage IV. There is rotation and horizontal adduction of the arm and, according to Wild, '. . . the outstanding trend disclosed by the movement types is change from movements in the anterio-posterior plane to movements largely in the horizontal plane, and from an unchanging base of support to left-foot-step forward' (Wild 1938, pp. 22–3).

Roberton's (1977a,b; 1978) major research thrust has been to validate overarm throwing sequences and to ascertain whether the throwing pattern progresses in an orderly fashion, or whether elements in the pattern develop in a different order for each child. She was of the opinion that if the elements for a pattern like throwing developed in a reliable and orderly fashion, then the stage hypothesis of motor development would be validated.

In another study a sequence was first hypothesized and then tested in a film study of 76 children (aged between 5 years and 9 years), who were observed for two to three consecutive years. As a test of the stage theory, she determined that children had to have a similar movement pattern for at least 50% of the trials. Stability of the sequence was evaluated by testing the children over a 2–3 year period and noting whether they progressed according to the hypothesized sequence and did not skip any of the categories (Roberton, 1978).

Roberton (1978) found that the action of the forearm and upperarm was stable from one trial to the next and changes occurred in the order that she had predicted. Pelvic-spinal categories, however, did not change in the expected fashion and so did not meet the specified criteria. She also noted that many of the children's movement pattern components, and particularly the pelvic-spinal component, did not change over the 2–3 year period. These data according to Roberton, raise questions about stage theory in relation to motor development, even though it has been a dominant developmental theory for at least 50 years. Further data of interest from this study were that only 43% of the children showed progressive changes in arm action over the 2–3 year time period (Roberton, 1978). Of these, only 59% had reached a mature arm action even though early researchers (e.g., Wellman, 1937) claimed most children reached mature patterns by 6 years of age.

Another issue in the literature that has been debated for many years, is the effect of inherent versus learnt factors in the throwing patterns (Dusenberry, 1952; Hicks, 1930; Wild, 1938). In one study, for example, children (3 year olds, n = 3; 4 year olds, n = 18; 5 year olds, n = 18; and 6 year olds, n = 12) were required to throw a squash ball at a 4 ft (120 cm) wide target, which was moved along an 8 ft (240 cm) track, at a speed of 33 ft per second (10 m/s), and aim for the green bull's eye which was 7 inches (18 cm) wide. No significant difference was found between the group that practised the test once a week for eight weeks and the control group that only undertook the initial and final test. Hicks claimed that these results demonstrate that improvement in throwing skill is due more to maturation (i.e. inherent) factors, rather than practice.

Wild (1938) was also of the opinion that maturation factors were important in the basic movement patterns, but she claimed that from about 6 years of age learning and practice influenced the level of skill in a movement pattern. Experiential factors, according to Wild, may also partly explain the performance and movement pattern superiority of boys in comparison to girls.

This particular interest of whether improvement in throwing is due to instruction (i.e. learning) in the skill of throwing, rather than improvement due to maturation factors prompted another study (Dusenberry, 1952). This study tested 56 children (aged from 3 to 7 years), who were divided into a experimental and control group, on the basis of age, gender and the distance they threw the ball. The children in the experimental group received practice sessions twice a week for three weeks. Instruction was found to influence stance and this was the major change observed in the control group, since most of the children at the end of the experiment stood with their opposite foot forward, which allowed greater body rotation and increased distance thrown. No noticeable difference occurred in the arm action or use of the fingers, which were apparently unaffected by instruction. Boys had a more mature pattern and threw further on the initial and final tests. Furthermore, despite the fact that the 3 and 4 year olds in the control group did not improve, there was a marked improvement in the 5–6 year old group (Dusenberry, 1952). From the data it could be claimed that children of 4 years of age and under will not improve their throwing performance and there will be little change in basic movement patterns if children are given only brief periods of practice.

In another study investigating the effects of learning, two weeks of throwing practice (120 min in total) was given to 45 kindergarten children who were randomly divided by gender into experimental and control groups (Halverson *et al.*, 1977). The first control group received a movement programme which did not include throwing practice; there also was a second control group that did not participate in any movement programme. Horizontal ball velocities were measured for each child. The authors found no significant difference in horizontal ball velocity between the experimental group that had extra throwing practice and the two groups that had no extra throwing practice (Halverson *et al.*, 1977). These results once again suggest that little if any change occurs in throwing patterns in young children, even with a short period of intensive practice.

A follow-up study of the levels of maturity reached in throwing patterns in older children (mean age 12 years 11 months, boys; and 13 years, girls), was conducted by Halverson, Roberton and Langendorfer (1982). The children had participated in an earlier study by Roberton (1978). They were assessed on the movement components of the upper arm, action of the forearm and the trunk. It was found that the children's modal categories for the three movement components were highly consistent.

In addition, the data showed that few of the girls had a mature trunk action; 12% had a mature forearm action and 20% had a mature humeral action. In contrast 31% of the boys had a mature trunk action, 41% a mature forearm action and 82% had an advanced humeral action (Halverson, Roberton and Langendorfer, 1982). A questionnaire, given to the children, revealed that the boys had participated in more activities which had enabled them to practice the overarm throw, than the girls. The data from this study are of additional interest because it clearly shows that boys, even though they had extended practice, had not attained the mature level in their throwing patterns by 13 years of age. Furthermore, since girls had less mature levels than boys at the same age, some of this delay could reflect, in part, lack of practice in this skill. These results did indicate, though, that the extended practice of the boys did result in them acquiring more mature movement patterns than those exhibited by the girls.

Summary of changes in the throwing pattern

Once the basic throwing pattern is acquired, changes usually occur in the upper body first, for example, the appearance of horizontal trunk rotation in the throwing arm and trunk on the same side of the body. Apart from this rotational movement the child still faces the target and there is little or no lower limb movement during the throwing pattern. The actual throw starts with a forward swing of the arm, and the object is then released from the hands (Espenchade and Eckert, 1980; O'Brien, 1991; Wickstrom, 1977, 1983; Wild, 1938). The arm action is similar to the previous developmental level except that the forearm is swung further in front of the body before the object is released. A unique characteristic of the next level of the throwing pattern is that the child steps forward on the leg, on the same side as the throwing arm (unilateral pattern) (O'Brien, 1991; Wickstrom, 1977, 1983; Wild, 1938).

In the mature pattern the body is side-on to the target in preparation for the start of the throw. At the start of the throw the weight is rocked onto the back foot, on the same side of the body as the throwing arm, the arm is swung backwards with marked trunk rotation, the humerus is parallel to the ground and the elbow is held at right angles. The throw is initiated by a step forward on the front foot (opposite foot to the moving arm), and rotation of the upper trunk towards the front foot. The arm is then whipped forward at right angles to impart maximum velocity to the thrown object (O'Brien, 1988, 1991; Wickstrom, 1983).

Figure 5.5 (a–d) (pp. 138–41) comprises of a pictorial summary of the development of the throwing pattern.

CONCLUSION ON FINDINGS FROM THE LITERATURE REVIEW

The literature review of the fundamental movement patterns has established that there is an orderly progression within each of the intratask skills of walking, running, jumping, catching and throwing. This progression appears to be based on components from the previous developmental level of the skill. Furthermore, any changes which do occur may not all be present in each child at one time. It does appear though, that there is sufficient similarity in sequential progression through the developmental levels in different groups of children, for many characteristic patterns to be regarded as stable and, as this terminology implies, representative of a level of development.

Observational criteria of the movement patterns are important to workers in the field. They are also important as the basis for establishing whether children with identified motor problems progress through the movement patterns in a similar way to normally developing children. Therefore, methodological and research procedures, together with suggested developmental movement sequences are considered in the next chapter.

REFERENCES

Bril, B. and Breneire, Y. (1992) Postural requirements and progression velocity in young walkers. *Journal of Motor Behavior*, **24**, 105–16.

Brown, J.M.M. and Parker, A.W. (1992) Comparison of gait in five- to seven-year old children. *Journal of Human Movement Studies*, **22**, 101–15.

Burnett, C.N. and Johnson, E.W. (1971a) Development of gait in childhood, Part 1: Method. *Developmental Medicine and Child Neurology*, **13**, 196–206.

Burnett, C.N. and Johnson, E.W. (1971b) Development of gait in childhood: Part 2. *Developmental Medicine and Child Neurology*, **13**, 207–15.

Clark, J.E. and Whitall, J. (1989) Changing patterns of locomotion: from walking to skipping, in *Development of Posture and Gait Across the Life Span*, (eds. M.H. Woollacott and A. Shumway-Cook), University of Southern California, Columbia, pp. 128–51.

Cratty, B.J. (1979) *Perceptual and Motor Development in Infants and Young Children*, Prentice-Hall, Englewood Cliffs, NJ.

Davis, K. (1988) Developmental differences in the use of peripheral vision during catching performance. *Journal of Motor Behaviour*, **20**, 39–51.

Dusenberry, L. (1952) A study of the effects of training in ball throwing by children ages three to seven. *Research Quarterly*, **23**, 9–14.

Espenchade, A.S. and Eckert, H.M. (1980) *Motor Development*. Charles E. Merrill, Columbus, OH.

Fischer, K.W. and Lazerson, A. (1984) *Human Development*, W.H. Freeman, New York.

Fortney, V.L. (1983) The kinematics and kinetics of the running pattern of two-, four- and six-year-old children. *Research Quarterly for Exercise and Sport*, **54**, 126–35.

Gesell, A. (1973) *The First Five Years of Life*, Methuen, London.

Halverson, H.M. (1931) An experimental study of prehension in infants by means of systematic cinema records. *Genetic Psychology Monographs*, **10**, 107–285.

Halverson, L.E. and Roberton, M.A. (1978) The effects of instruction on overhand throwing development in children, in *Psychology of Motor Behaviour and Sport*, (eds G.C. Roberts and K.M. Newell), Human Kinetics, Champaign, IL, pp. 258–69.

Halverson, L.E., Roberton, M.A. and Langendorfer, S. (1982) Development of the overarm throw: movement and ball velocity changes by seventh grade. *Research Quarterly for Exercise and Sport*, **53**, 198–205.

Halverson, L. and Williams, K. (1985) Developmental sequences for hopping over distance a prelongitudinal screening. *Research Quarterly for Exercise and Sport*, **56**, 37–44.

Halverson, L.E., Roberton, M.A., Safrit, M.J. and Roberts, T.W. (1977) Effects of guided practice on overhand-throw ball velocities of kindergarten children. *Research Quarterly*, **48**, 311–18.

Hellebrandt, F.A., Rarick, L., Glassow, R. and Carns, M.L. (1961) Physiological analysis of basic motor skills: 1. Growth and development of jumping. *American Journal of Physical Medicine*, **40**, 14–25.

Hicks, J.A. (1930) The acquisition of motor skills in young children: a study of the effects of practice in throwing at a moving target. *Child Development*, **1**, 90–105.

McClenaghan, B.A. and Gallahue, D.L. (1978) *Fundamental Movement: A Developmental and Remedial Approach*, W.B. Saunders, Philadelphia.

McGraw, M.B. (1966) *The Neuromuscular Maturation of the Human Infant*. Hafner, New York.

Morris, A.M., Williams, J.M., Atwater, A.E. and Wilmore, J.H. (1982) Age and sex differences in motor performance of 3 through 6 year old children. *Research Quarterly for Exercise and Sport*, **53**, 214–21.

O'Brien, C.C. (1988) *Motor Development in Clumsy, Intellectually Disabled and Down's Syndrome Children: A Comparative Study*. Unpublished PhD thesis, University of Queensland.

O'Brien, C.C. (1991) *Motor Development in Young Children*, V.R. Ward, Government Printer, Brisbane.

O'Brien, C.C. and Ziviani, J. (1991) *Fine Motor Development and Young Children*, V.R. Ward, Government Printer, Brisbane.

O'Brien, C.C. and Hayes, A. (1989) Motor development in early childhood of clumsy, intellectually disabled and Down's Syndrome children. *The ACHPER National Journal*, **124**, 15–19.

Phillips, S.J., Clark, J.E. and Petersen, R.D. (1985) Developmental differences in standing long jump takeoff parameters. *Journal of Human Movement Studies*, **11**, 75–87.
Rarick, G.L. (1982) Descriptive research and process-oriented explanations of the motor development of children, in *The Development of Movement Control and Co-ordination*, (eds J.A.S. Kelso and J.E. Clark), John Wiley, Chichester, pp. 275–91.
Roberton, M.A. (1977a) Stability of stage categorizations across trials: implications for the 'Stage Theory' of overarm throw development. *Journal of Human Movement Studies*, **3**, 49–59.
Roberton, M.A. (1977b) Stability of stage categorizations in motor development, in *Psychology of Motor Behavior and Sport* (eds M. Landers and R.W. Christina), Human Kinetics, Champaign, IL, pp. 494–506.
Roberton, M.A. (1978) Longitudinal evidence for developmental stages in the forceful overarm throw. *Journal of Human Movement Studies*, **4**, 167–75.
Roberton, M.A. (1984) Changing motor patterns during childhood, in *Motor Development During Childhood and Adolescence*, (ed J.R. Thomas), Burgess, Minneapolis, pp. 48–90.
Seefeldt, V. (1979) Developmental motor patterns: implications for elmentary school physical education, in *Psychology of Motor Behavior and Sport*, (eds C.H. Nadeau, W.R. Halliwell, K.M. Newell and G.C. Roberts), Human Kinetics, Champaign, IL, pp. 314–23.
Seefeldt, V. and Haubenstricker, J. (1982) Patterns, phases or stages: an analytical model for the study of developmental movement, in *The Development of Movement Control and Co-ordination*, (eds J.A.S. Kelso and J.E. Clark), John Wiley, Chichester, pp. 309–18.
Shirley, M.M. (1931) *The First Two Years*. University of Minnesota Press, Minneapolis.
Sinclair, C.B. (1973) *Movement of the Young Child: Ages Two to Six* Charles E. Merrill, Columbus, OH.
Smyth, M.M. and Marriott, A.M. (1982) Vision and proprioception in simple catching. *Journal of Motor Behavior*, **14**, 143–52.
Strohmeyer, H.S., Williams, K. and Schaub-George, D. (1991) Developmental sequences for catching a small ball: a prelongitudinal screening. *Research Quarterly for Exercise and Sport*, **62**, 257–66.
Sutherland, D.H., Olsen, R., Cooper, L. and Woo, S.L.Y. (1980) The development of mature gait. *The Journal of Bone and Joint Surgery*, **62A**, 336–53.
Thelen, E., Ulrich, B.D. and Jensen, J.L. (1989) The developmental origins of locomotion, in *Development of Posture and Gait Across the Life Span*, (eds M.H. Woollacott and A. Shumway-Cook), University of Southern California, Columbia, pp. 25–47.
Wellman, B.L. (1937) Motor achievement of preschool children. *Childhood Education*, **13**, 311–16.
Wheelwright, E.F., Minns, R.A., Law, H.T. and Elton, R.A. (1993)

Temporal and spatial parameters of gait in children 1: Normal control data. *Developmental Medicine and Child Neurology*, **35**, 102–113.

Whiting, H.T.A. (1969) *Acquiring Ball Skill, a Psychological Interpretation*, G. Bell, London.

Whiting, H.T.A., Savelsbergh, G.J.P. and Faber, C.M. (1988) 'Catch' questions and incomplete answers, in *Cognition and Action in Skilled Behaviour* (eds A.M. Colley and J.R. Beech), North Holland, Elsevier Science, Amsterdam, pp. 257–71.

Wickstrom, R.L. (1977) Fundamental motor patterns, Lea & Febiger, Philadelphia.

Wickstrom, R.L. (1983) Fundamental motor patterns (3rd edn.), Lea & Febiger, Philadelphia.

Wild, M.R. (1938) The behavior pattern of throwing and some observations concerning its course of development in children. *Research Quarterly*, **9**, 20–4.

Winter, D.A. (1983) Biomechanical motor patterns in normal walking. *Journal of Motor Behavior*, **15**, 302–30.

Zanone, P.G. (1990) Tracking with and without target in 6- to 15-year-old boys. *Journal of Motor Behavior*. **22**, 225–49.

Zimmerman, H.M. (1956) Characteristic likenesses and differences between skilled and non-skilled performance of the standing broad jump. *Research Quarterly*, **27**, 352–62.

5

Sequences of fundamental movement patterns

This chapter examines methodological and research issues pertinent to studying fundamental movement patterns. Before studying sequential progression in fundamental movement patterns it is first necessary to discuss some of the methodological and conceptual issues which have been debated by researchers in this area. The discussion of methodological issues includes consideration of the way in which other researchers have studied movement patterns and the methodology for developing movement sequences suitable for assessing changes in motor impaired children's movement patterns.

OVERVIEW

In deriving developmental sequences, early researchers used either direct observational methods or conducted observational studies on previously filmed data (Dusenberry, 1952; Gesell, 1973; Hicks, 1930; Wild, 1938). Most of these researchers had subjectively listed observational information on the spatial–temporal organization of the movement pattern, as well as age-related changes in the organization of the patterns. There was a general consensus among the researchers that the fundamental movement patterns become progressively more complex with increased age. Moreover, the notion of stage theory as an explanation of developmental changes in the sequences so dominated the developmental literature that many authors did not question its assumptions (e.g. Ames and

Ilg, 1966; Gesell, 1973). Recently, however, the major conceptual issue in the study of fundamental movement patterns has focused on whether the entire movement pattern changes abruptly from one level to another (stage theory). Or, alternatively whether there is a progression of the units of movement within each pattern, in terms of interlimb and bodily changes. Two researchers in particular, Roberton and Seefeldt (and their associates) have debated this issue and their differing positions will be discussed next.

Roberton (1977a,b, 1978) questioned the assumption that children's total movement pattern configurations change abruptly from one level to another. Instead after further studies of the throwing pattern (Halverson, Roberton and Langendorfer, 1982; Roberton and Di Rocco, 1981), she concluded that age-related, or developmental changes in the fundamental movement patterns are more likely to be observed in the components (called elements in this book) that make up the movement patterns. She developed a model in which some of the components change more rapidly than others (Roberton, 1984).

In contrast, Seefeldt (1979) has taken a more global approach to fundamental movement pattern development. He is of the opinion that total body configuration changes abruptly from one level to the next as a result of more efficient movement. This is the result of application of better biomechanical principles and to the incorporation of more complex movements in the subroutines, such as a greater range of movement and better positioning of body segments for production of maximum force. Another reason for classifying fundamental movement patterns according to total body configurations, is because a system which classifies children's total movement patterns can be used by teachers and professionals in the field to identify levels of development in children's movement sequences (Seefeldt, 1979).

Despite their divergent opinions Seefeldt and Haubenstricker (1982) agree with Roberton's (1977a,b, 1978) claim that not all subroutines, or components of a subroutine, within an intratask movement sequence develop at the same rate. As a consequence, children at similar levels of development will appear different from other children in the group, because of different rates of progress in the different body segments which contribute to the fundamental movement pattern. Nevertheless, on the basis of filmed data collected longitudinally on children aged from 1 to 12 years, Seefeldt and Haubenstricker believe that there is sufficient cohesion between subroutines at a particular developmental level to justify classifying the movement pattern as belonging to a particular level of development which is distinct from other levels.

The authors of this book are of the opinion that provided there is a hierarchy of developmental progression, it really does not matter whether the progression is classified into components of development within each movement pattern, or levels of development. It is the verbal descriptions of the fundamental movement patterns that are important because they enable visualization of development and identification of variations from the normal progression.

Since fundamental movement patterns have the potential to provide valuable information about levels of development, as well as being an important observational tool, it was considered necessary to devise a method to standardize the sequences for walking, running, jumping, catching and throwing to be used in the study reported in this book. The method which was used is outlined in the following section.

DEVELOPMENT AND VALIDATION OF MOVEMENT SEQUENCES

Early researchers (e.g., Ames and Ilg, 1966; Hicks, 1930; Shirley, 1931; Wellman, 1937; Wild, 1938) used observational techniques and classified children into stages on the basis of the number of children who progressed through a particular movement pattern. Some of the early studies were cross-sectional, some longitudinal, and others a mixture of both. Similar cross-sectional, longitudinal or mixed designs are still used (e.g. Burnett and Johnson, 1971a,b; Halverson, Roberton and Langendorfer, 1982; Seefeldt and Haubenstricker, 1982; Sinclair 1973).

The design and methodology used in this book to derive the movement sequences are the ones proposed by Roberton, Williams and Langendorfer (1980) for prelongitudinal screening of motor development sequences. According to these authors 'one of the tasks of the developmental researcher . . . is to identify those skills or skill groupings which show sequences and describe the response order' (p. 724).

The screening procedure that was used in the study reported later in the chapter, involves the following steps. First, a hypothesized sequence of skill development is compiled that is derived from an extensive literature review and observations by the researcher. Second, a cross-sectional study is conducted to verify that there is an age-related progression in the proposed sequence. The verification of the sequence depends on whether more of the less mature children's movement patterns are in the lower levels of the sequence and whether the movement patterns of the more mature children are in the higher levels of the proposed sequence. This means that there is an age-related decrease in frequency of children at the lower levels, with an increase in frequency of children at a higher level. (It must be remembered that in an initial prelongitudinal screening cross-sectional study, age is substituted for development, even though development is not necessarily synonymous with increased age.) Third, should the prelongitudinal study confirm that the selected sample of children does tend to progress in the proposed developmental order, then the sequence warrants validation by a longitudinal study (Roberton, Williams and Langendorfer, 1980).

The literature review for the first step in the above procedure has been reported in Chapter 4. The proposed sequences have been developed from the literature search and have been trialled on normally developing children (O'Brien, 1988, 1994; O'Brien and Hayes, 1989). These steps resulted in the sequences that are tabulated in this chapter (Tables 5.1–5.5), and the cross-sectional study of these sequences also is reported. A prelongitudinal screening procedure was considered important because the authors are aware of very few relevant developmental research studies which examine all the fundamental movement patterns in normally developing and exceptional children.

There are, however, some studies known to the authors on single movement patterns, for example, on the walking pattern of children with Down syndrome (Parker and Bronks, 1980; Parker, Bronks and Snyder, 1986) and on the temporal and spatial parameters of pathological gait in children

(Wheelwright *et al.*, 1993), another on the throwing pattern of intellectually disabled children (Roberton and Di Rocco, 1981) and one on the jumping coordination patterns of mildly intellectually disabled children (DiRocco, Clark and Phillips, 1987). These studies highlighted differences in individual fundamental patterns between motor impaired and normally developing children. All these studies found delays or differences in the fundamental movement patterns of motor impaired children.

THE HYPOTHESIZED DEVELOPMENTAL SEQUENCES

As a result of the literature search and screening procedures (O'Brien, 1988), hypothesized developmental sequences in normal children were compiled for the fundamental movement patterns of walking, running, jumping, catching and throwing. Each movement pattern was subdivided into the following elements: general body appearance, upper body and limbs, lower body and limbs, basis of the movement pattern and additional criteria. These sequences are summarized in Tables 5.1–5.5 and Figures 5.1–5.5.

These Fundamental Movement Pattern check-lists were used in a study which is reported in the next section of the chapter. (For a summary of the method, procedure and results, refer to Appendix B.)

A STUDY OF THE FUNDAMENTAL MOVEMENT PATTERNS OF CHILDREN WHO ARE DEVELOPING NORMALLY, CLUMSY, INTELLECTUALLY DISABLED OR HAVE DOWN SYNDROME

The Fundamental Movement Pattern check-lists (Tables 5.1–5.5) were used in this study. In each of the fundamental movement pattern profiles for the movement sequences of walking, running, jumping, catching and throwing, four different levels were devised. The lowest or least mature level was level one, and the highest or most mature level was level four. These levels were further subdivided into five different elements which were: general body appearance, upper body and limbs, lower body and limbs, basis of movement pattern and general criteria. The elements titled 'upper body and limbs'

Table 5.1 Fundamental movement pattern for walking

WALKING PROFILE

General body appearance

Level

1. Stiff movement: marked sideways sway: frequent falls.
2. Body held stiffly: some sway with each step: some falls.
3. Body held erect without tension: some sway with each step but little sideways or up and down movement.
4. Smooth, rhythmical, well-timed movements.

Upper body and limbs

Level

1. High rigid arm position: no armswing.
2. Arms held by side with little swing of trunk or arms.
3. Arms by side with some contralateral swing: one arm swings more than the other.
4. Arms and legs move in opposition to each other.

Lower body and limbs

Level

1. Flat foot contact with the ground: out-toeing of feet or marked in-toeing: stereotyped stepping action.
2. Elements of heel–toe foot contact with each step: moderate out-toeing or in-toeing: some ability to modify stepping action.

3. Heel–toe foot contact with each step: slight out-toeing or in-toeing: ability to modify action for different ground surfaces.
4. Smooth heel–toe transfer of weight: adaptation action.

Basis of movement pattern

Level

1. High bent knee stepping action: wide base of support and/or marked hip flexion.
2. Moderate bent knee stepping action: knee lock on ground contact with forward leg: moderate width base of support.
3. Double knee lock during two step phase (i.e. a knee lock of the forward leg after contact with the ground and on support leg during forward swing phase): base of support narrower than trunk.
4. Contralateral leg and arm action counteracts lateral rotation of the body: narrow base of support.

Additional criteria

Level

1. Asymmetrical leg action and/or inconsistent stride length.
2. Some asymmetry in leg action and/or stride length.
3. Symmetry in leg action and stride length.
4. Symmetry in leg and arm action.

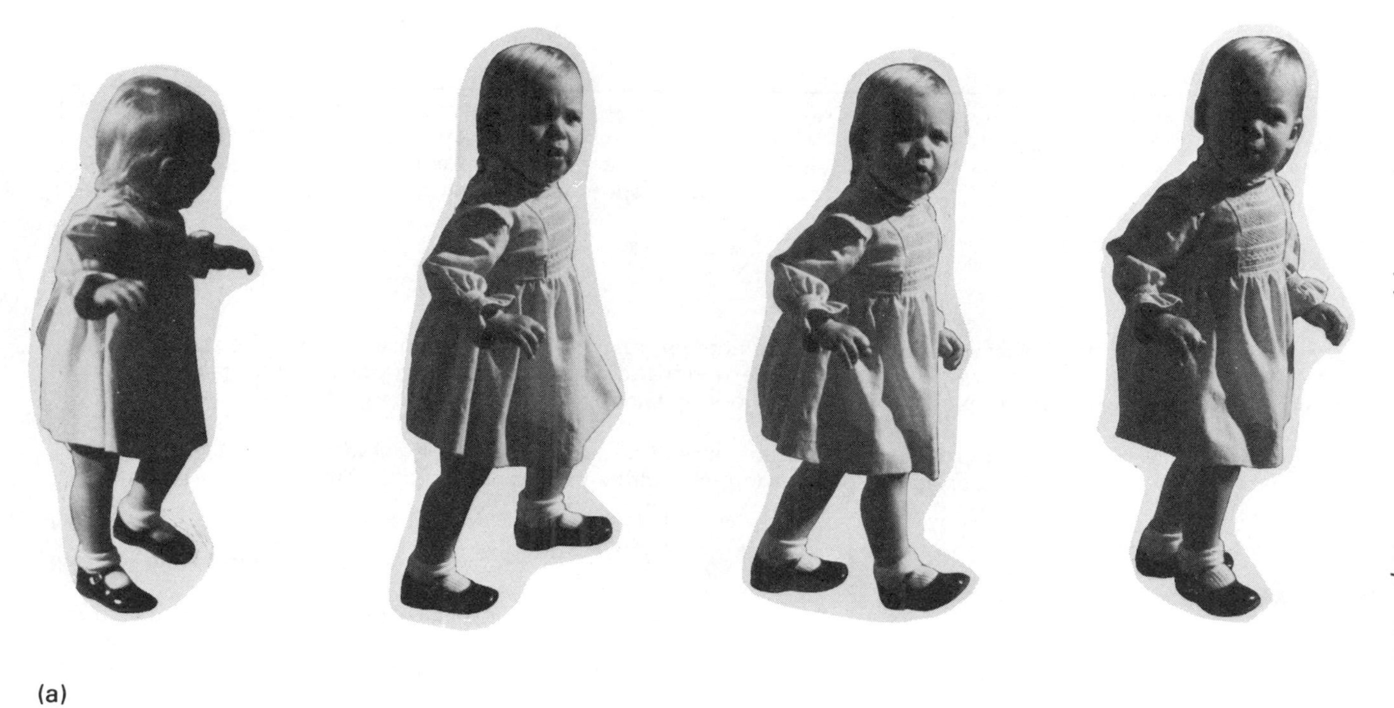

(a)

Figure 5.1 (a) Developmental levels of walking. Level 1.

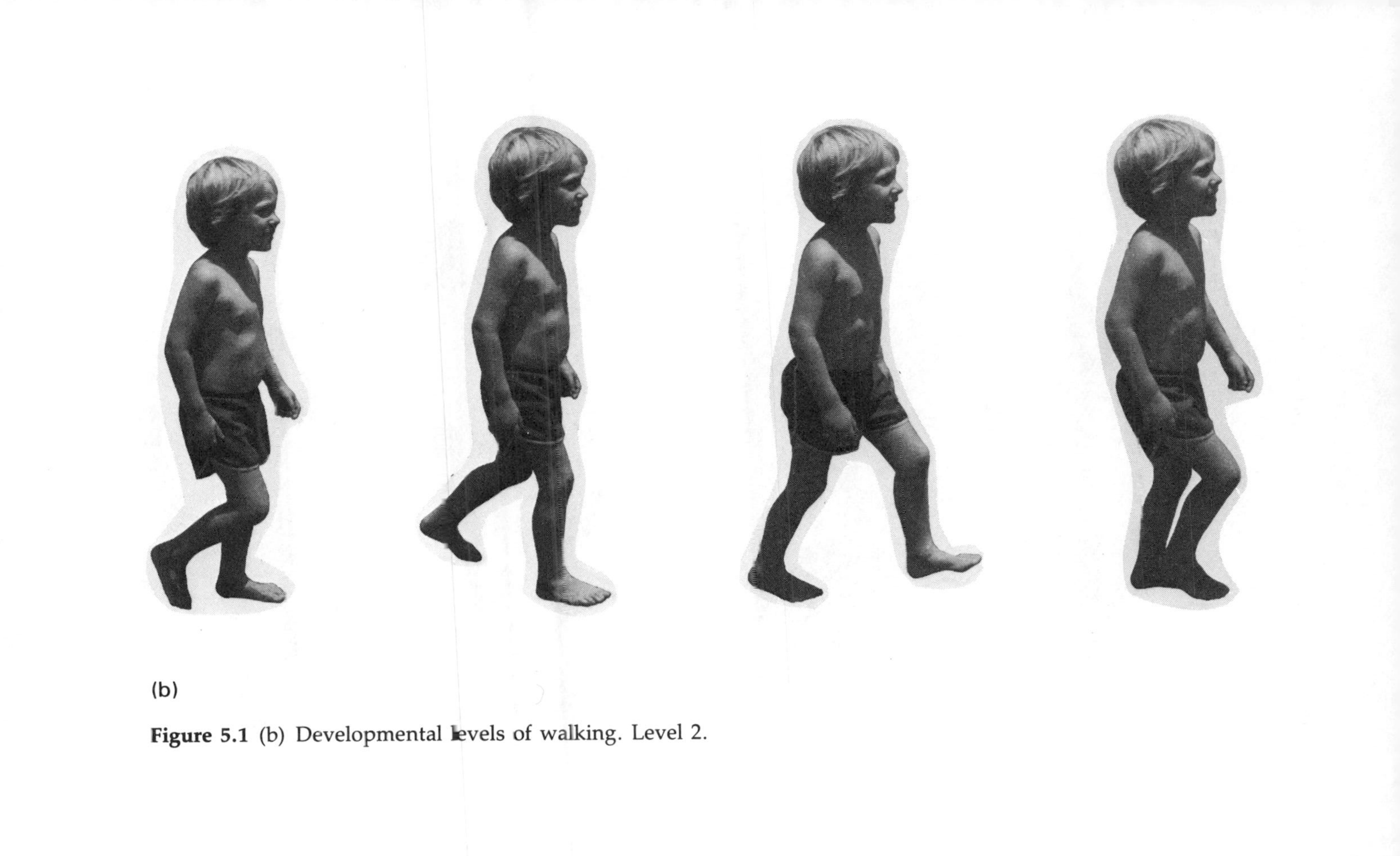

(b)

Figure 5.1 (b) Developmental levels of walking. Level 2.

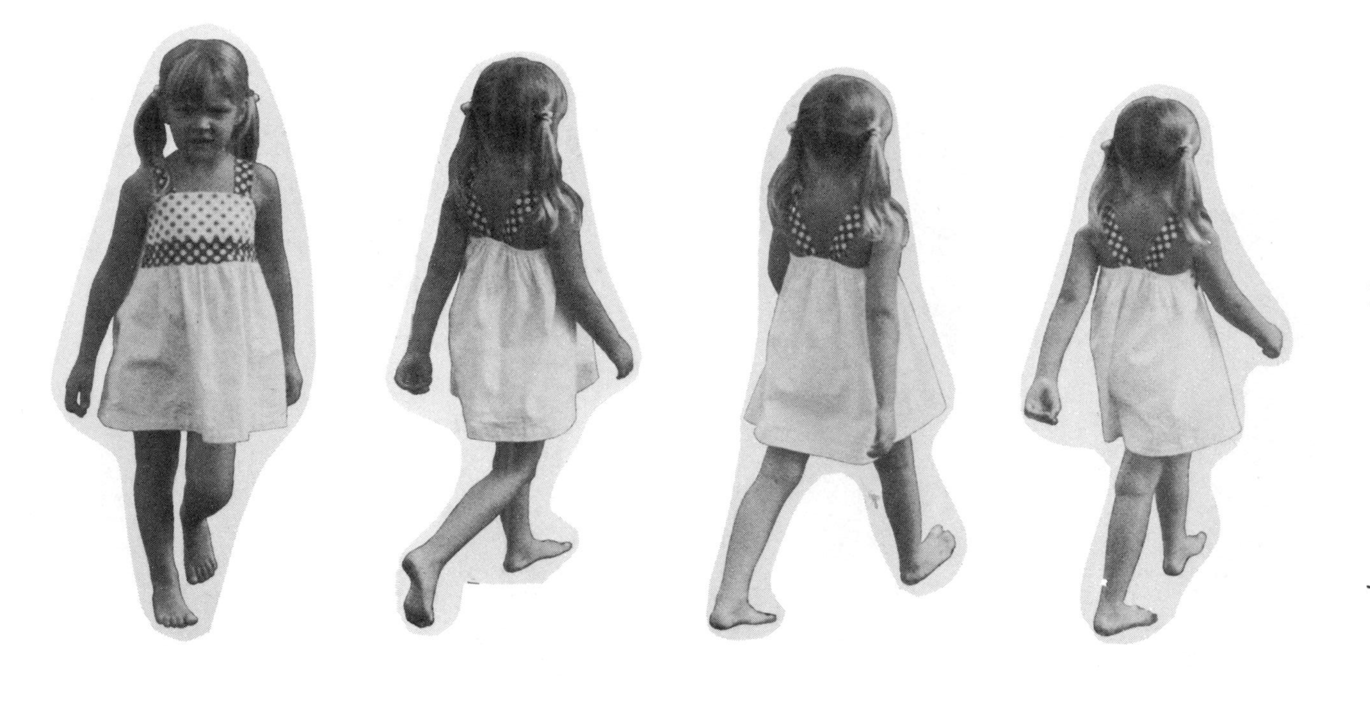

(c)

Figure 5.1 (c) Developmental levels of walking. Level 3.

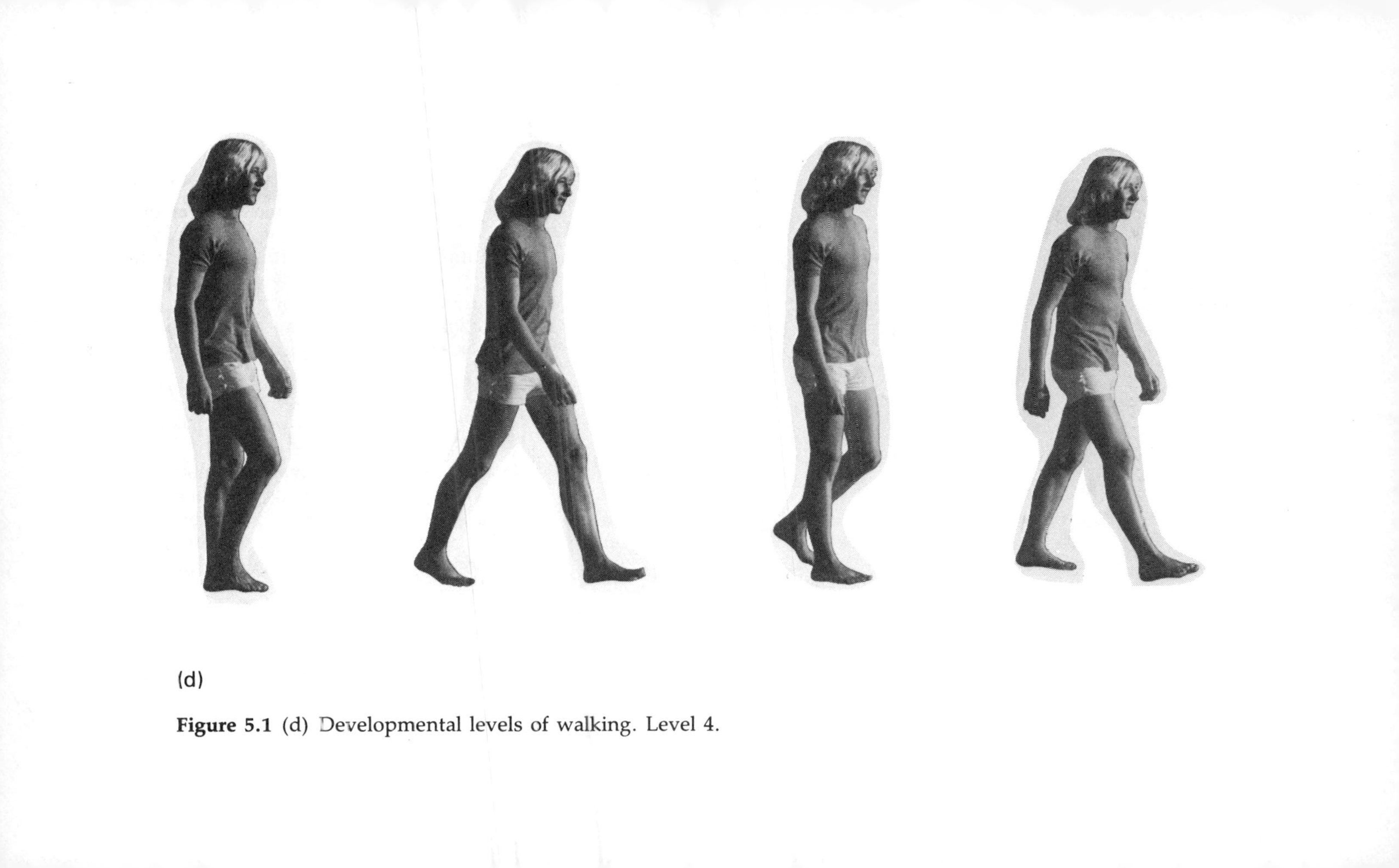

Figure 5.1 (d) Developmental levels of walking. Level 4.

Table 5.2 Fundamental movement pattern for running

RUNNING PROFILE

General body appearance

Level

1. Stiff, bouncy action: frequent falls.
2. Bouncy action: some falls especially when turning.
3. Smoother forward progression with less vertical than horizontal movement: can turn while running at a reasonable speed.
4. Fluent contralateral upper and lower limb movement.

Upper body and limbs

Level

1. High arm position: little or no arm swing.
2. Arms waist height or held straight: generally a restricted range of movement.
3. Asymmetrical arm action: one arm generally swung forward and backward with bent elbow, other swung from shoulder.
4. Arms and trunk movement symmetrical: arm swung forward and backward.

Lower body and limbs

Level

1. Small amounts of knee bend: feet remain close to ground with appearance of out-toeing or in-toeing: flat foot contact with ground.

2. More use of knee and ankle joint in the stepping action: still elements of flat foot contact with the ground.
3. Good use of knee, ankle and hip joint: front leg bent at angle of 90° during forward swing phase.
4. Complete straightening of the back leg at an angle of about 45° to the body, with high bent knee action in swing forward phase.

Basis of movement pattern

Level

1. No or a very brief airborne phase (generally one foot always in contact with the ground): limited range of joint movement in all limbs: wide base of support.
2. Some airborne phase, both feet off ground for a minimal time: greater range of joint movement especially in lower limbs: moderate base of support.
3. Moderate length airborne phase: good range of joint movements in lower limbs: increasing range in upper limbs: narrow base of support.
4. Extended airborne phase: marked flexion in joint movements in the lower limbs during the 'swinging' phase: upper limbs counterbalance the leg action and are swung backwards and forwards with a bent elbow.

Additional criteria

Level

1. No pelvic rotation: short and/or uneven stride length: may be symmetrical leg action and uneven stride length.
2. Some pelvic rotation: may be asymmetrical leg action.
3. Marked pelvic rotation with some children who have a powerful leg action: even, medium length stride.
4. Smooth pelvic rotation: even, long length stride.

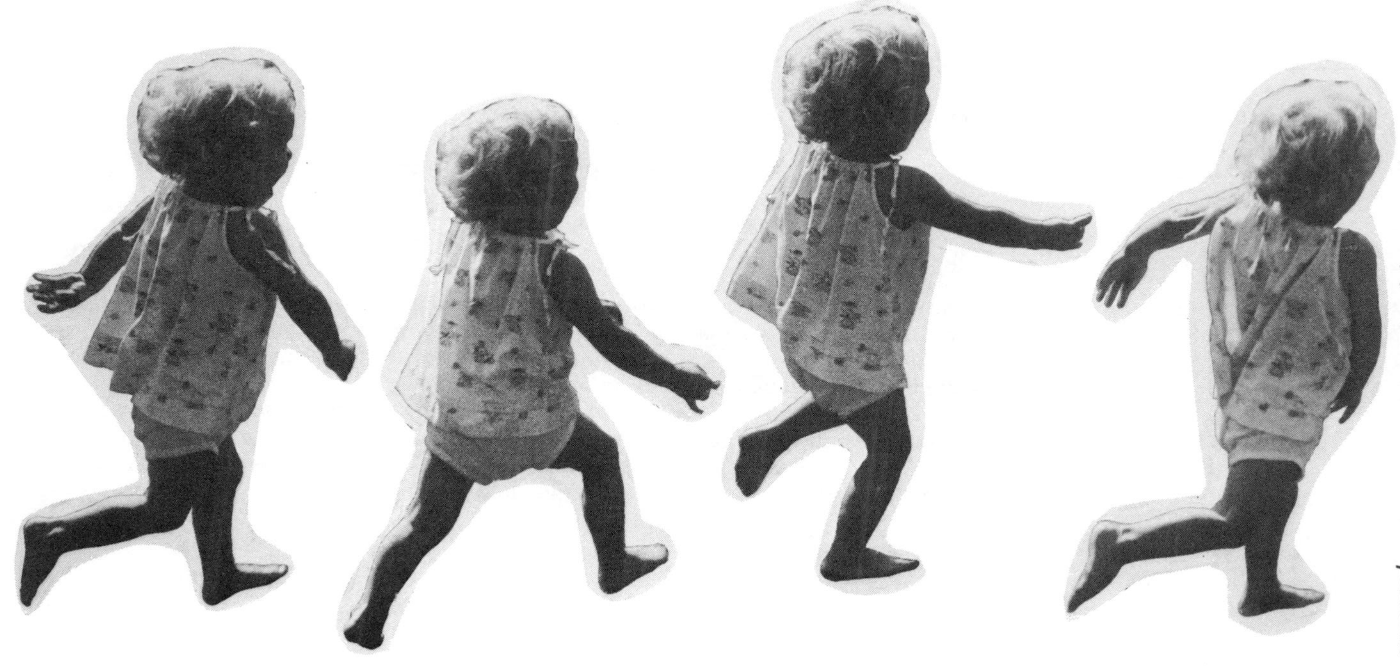

(a)

Figure 5.2 (a) Developmental levels of running. Level 1.

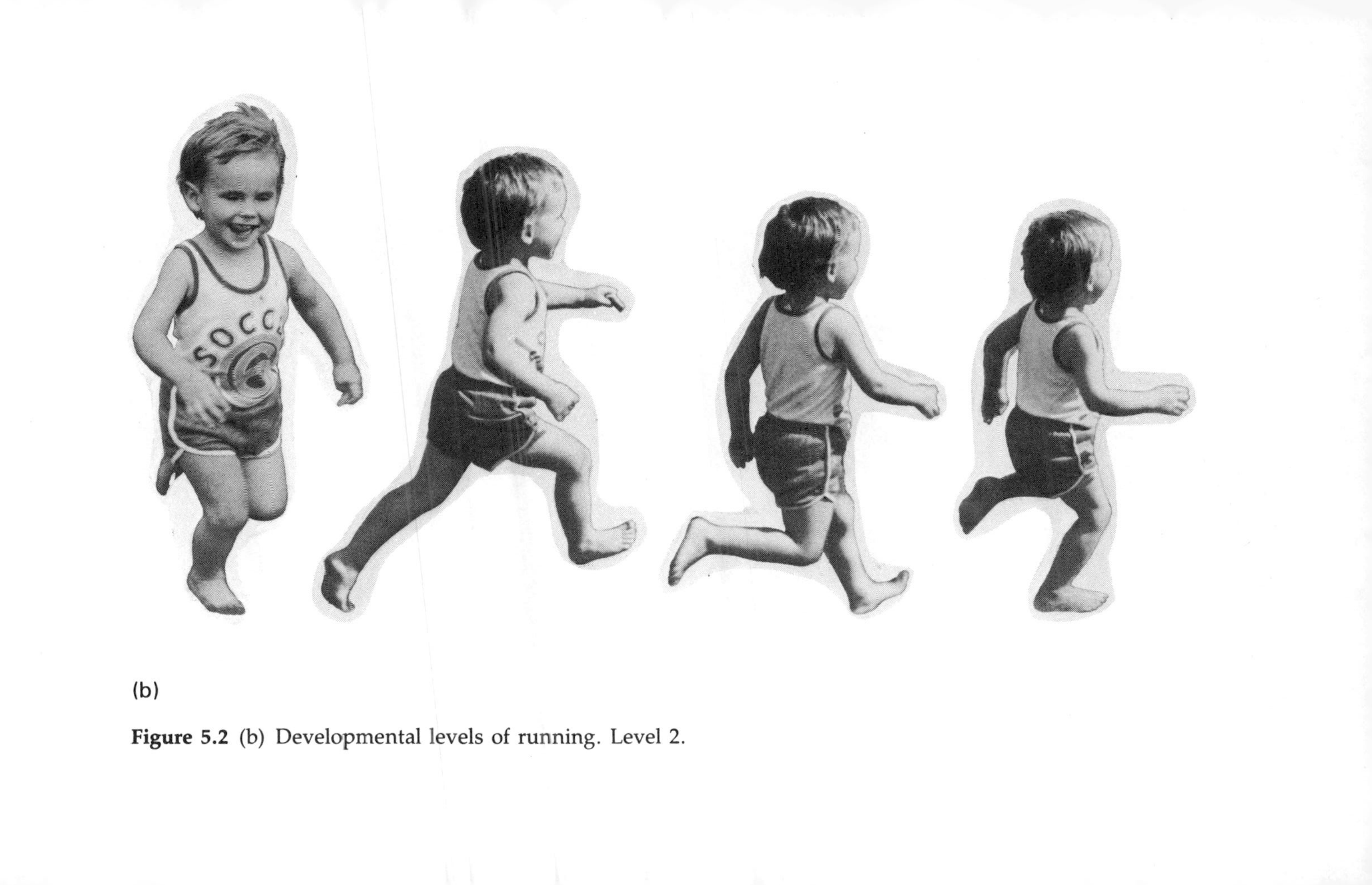

(b)

Figure 5.2 (b) Developmental levels of running. Level 2.

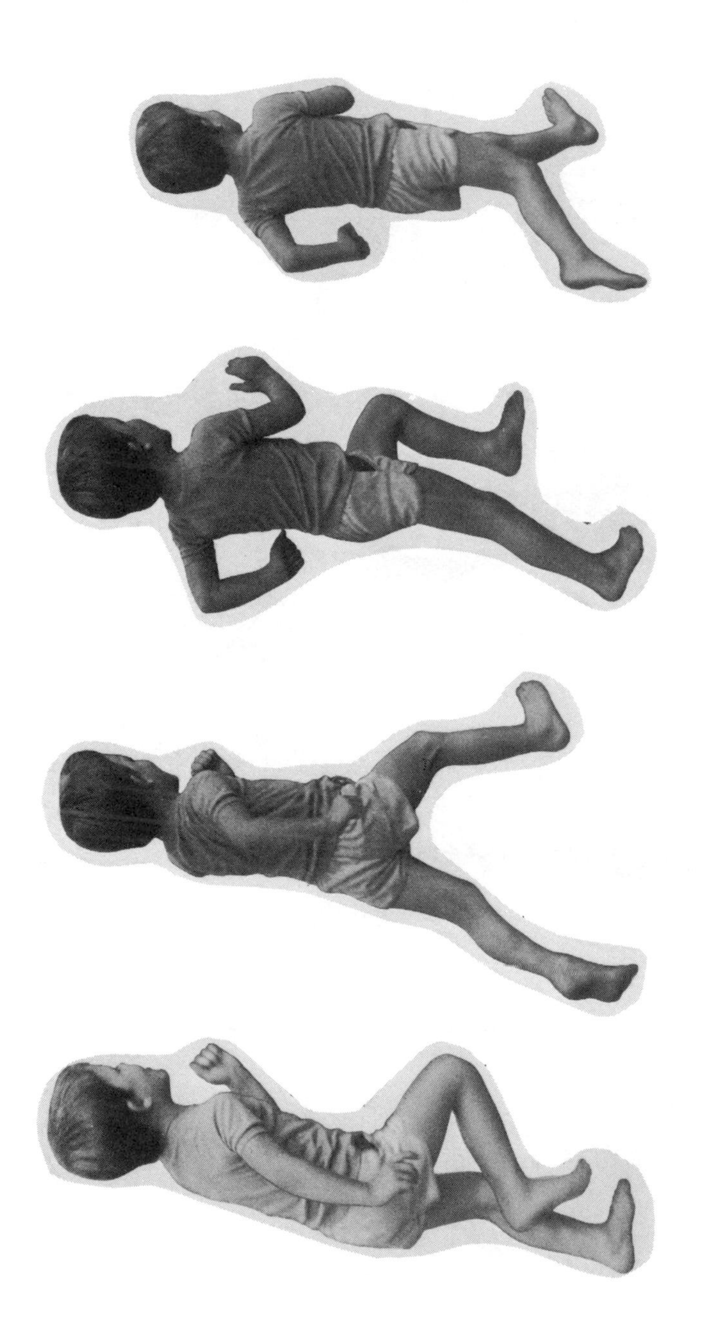

(c)

Figure 5.2 (c) Developmental levels of running. Level 3.

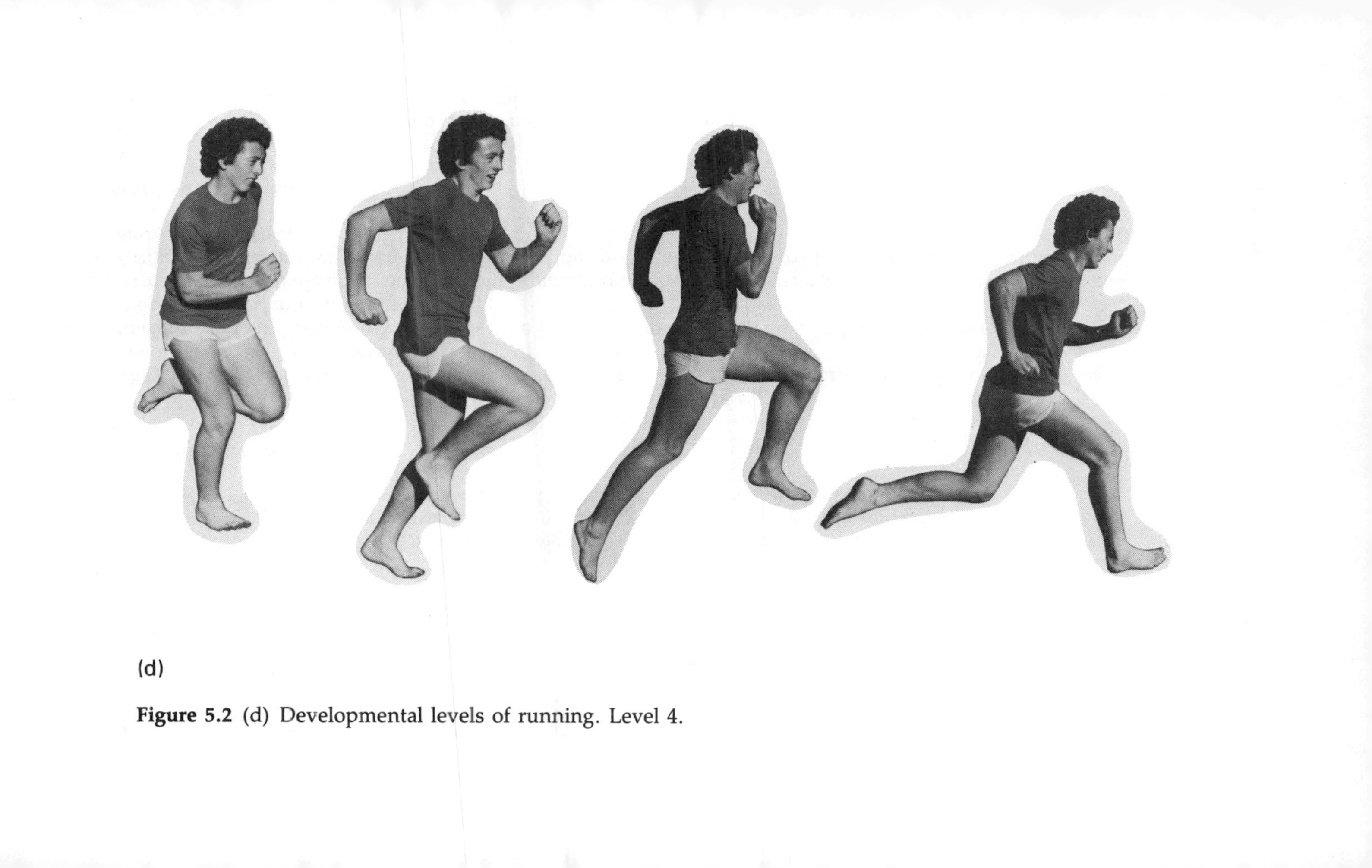

(d)

Figure 5.2 (d) Developmental levels of running. Level 4.

Table 5.3 Fundamental movement pattern for jumping

JUMPING PROFILE

General body appearance

Level

1. Body held upright and straight, before and during jump: jerky body movements.
2. Squat position before take-off: relatively straight position during jump: still jerky body movements.
3. Body and trunk inclination before take-off and during jump: less jerky body movement.
4. Complete synchronization of arms, legs and head: smooth, coordinated movements.

Upper body and limbs

Level

1. The beginnings of 'winging' arm action (both arms move slightly back during the airborne phase): little or no head movement: head controls action of upper body.
2. Marked 'winging' action of arms: still little head adjustment to changes in body position except for some preparation for and on landing.
3. Arms swing from side of the body to front horizontal or slightly sideways: head adjustment to changes in body position.
4. Arms swung back then extended above head during flight and forward to give a balanced landing: good head, and trunk control.

Lower body and limbs

Level

1. Stepping action before true jump, followed by straight leg jump: brief airborne phase: one foot take-off to one or two foot landing: poor lower limb control.

2. Legs straightened at take-off, bent backwards during flight and bent on landing: two foot take-off to poorly controlled landing.
3. Legs straightened on take-off, then bent backwards to about 90 degrees angle during flight, then swung forward for landing: long airborne phase: better lower limb control on take-off and landing.
4. Two foot take-off and landing: hitch kick in airborne phase: well-controlled lower limbs with two foot take-off to two foot landing.

Basis of movement pattern

Level

1. Jump performed by lower limbs: absence of trunk movement and fixed arm position.
2. After take-off arms are often swung backward and sideways to form 'birdwings': better use of lower limbs but still not symmetrical.
3. Some changes in leg and arm position during jump: good use of trunk and head.
4. Well coordinated take-off, flight and landing: symmetrical use of upper and lower limbs.

Additional criteria

Level

1. Non-effective use of the arms and upper body: no arm use, leg asymmetry: short jump.
2. Some use of trunk, head and arms: medium length jump.
3. Beginnings of opposition of arm and leg action and some head control: good length jump.
4. Effective use of arms, trunk and head to obtain maximum jumping distance.

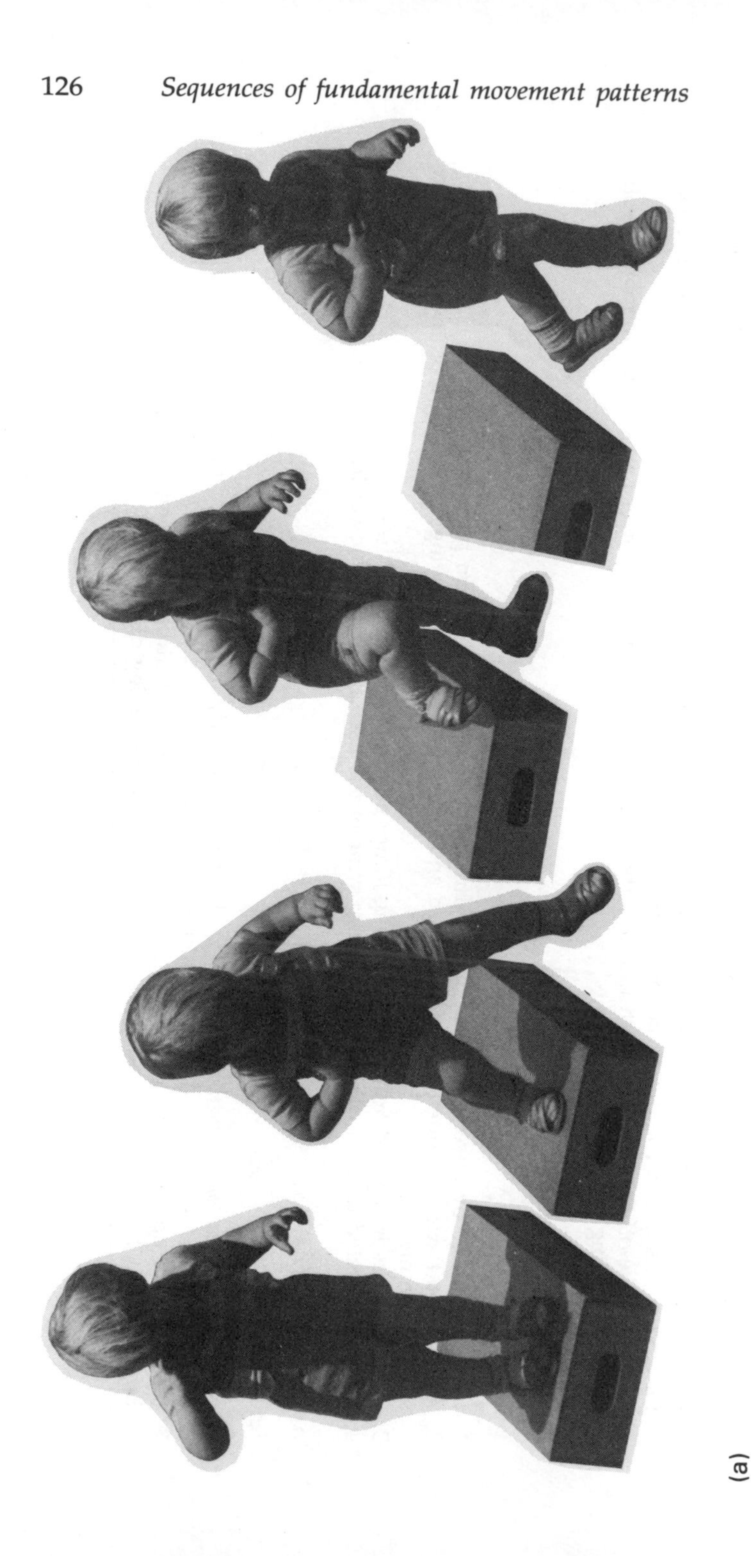

Figure 5.3 (a) Developmental levels of jumping. Level 1.

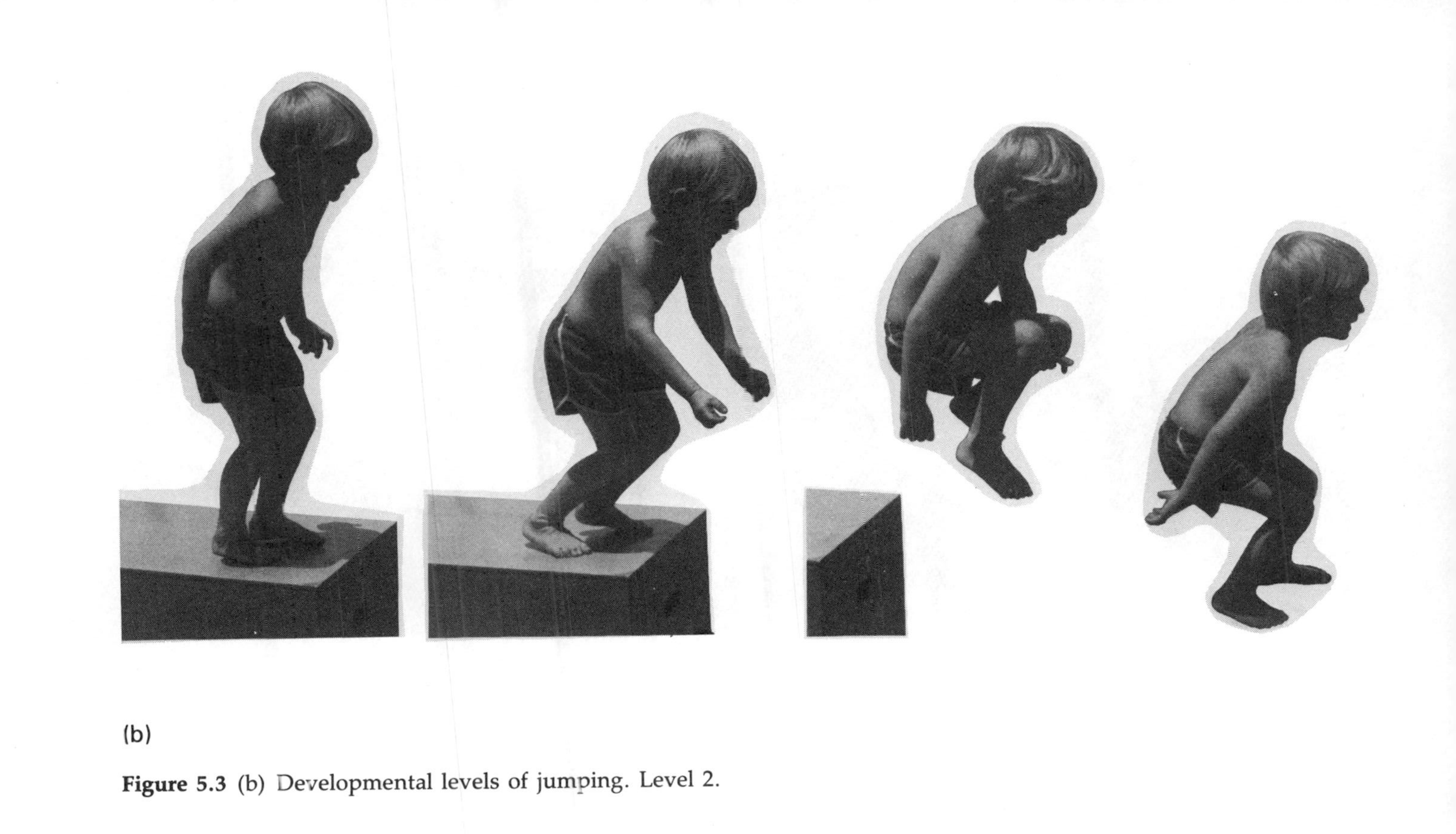

(b)

Figure 5.3 (b) Developmental levels of jumping. Level 2.

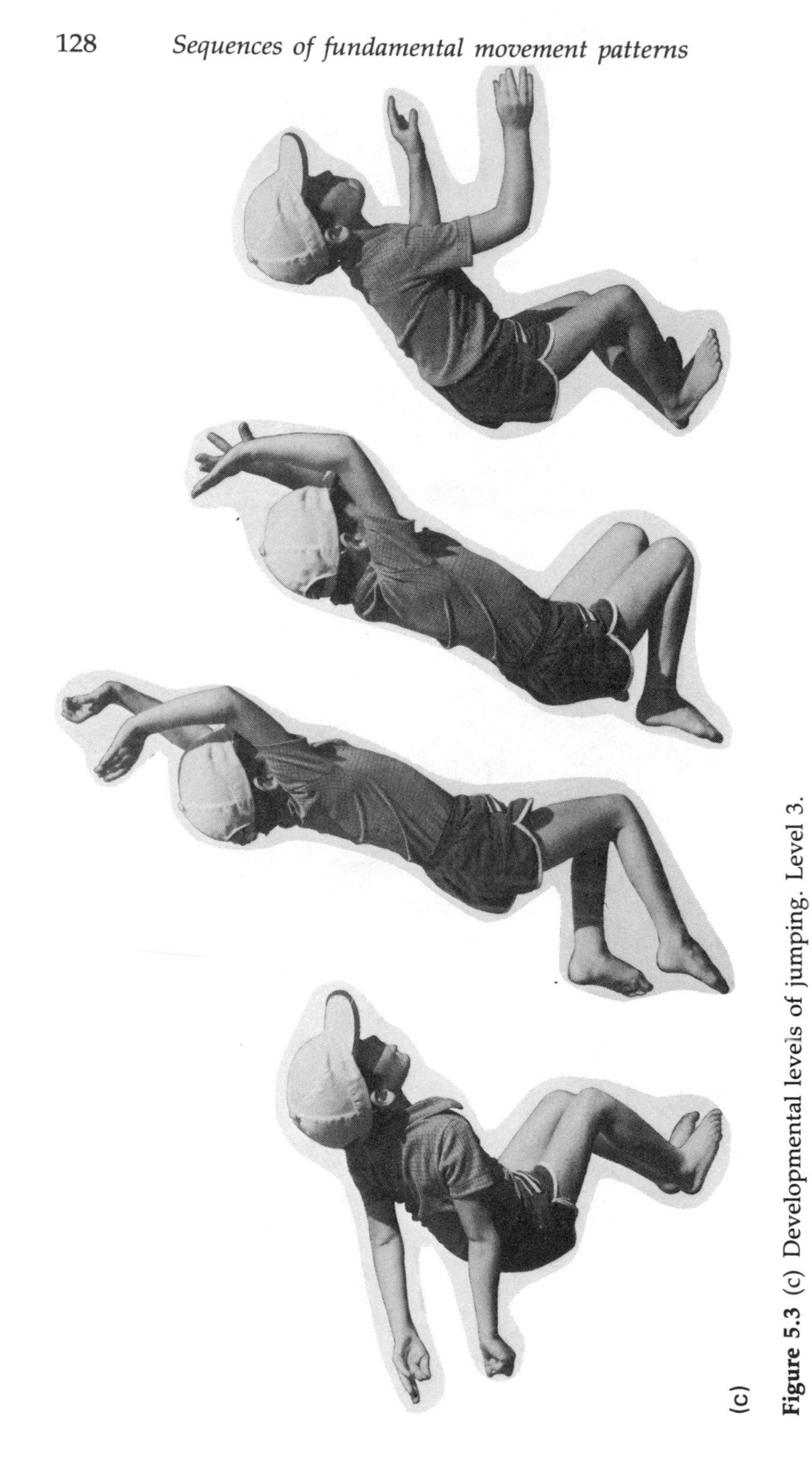

(c)

Figure 5.3 (c) Developmental levels of jumping. Level 3.

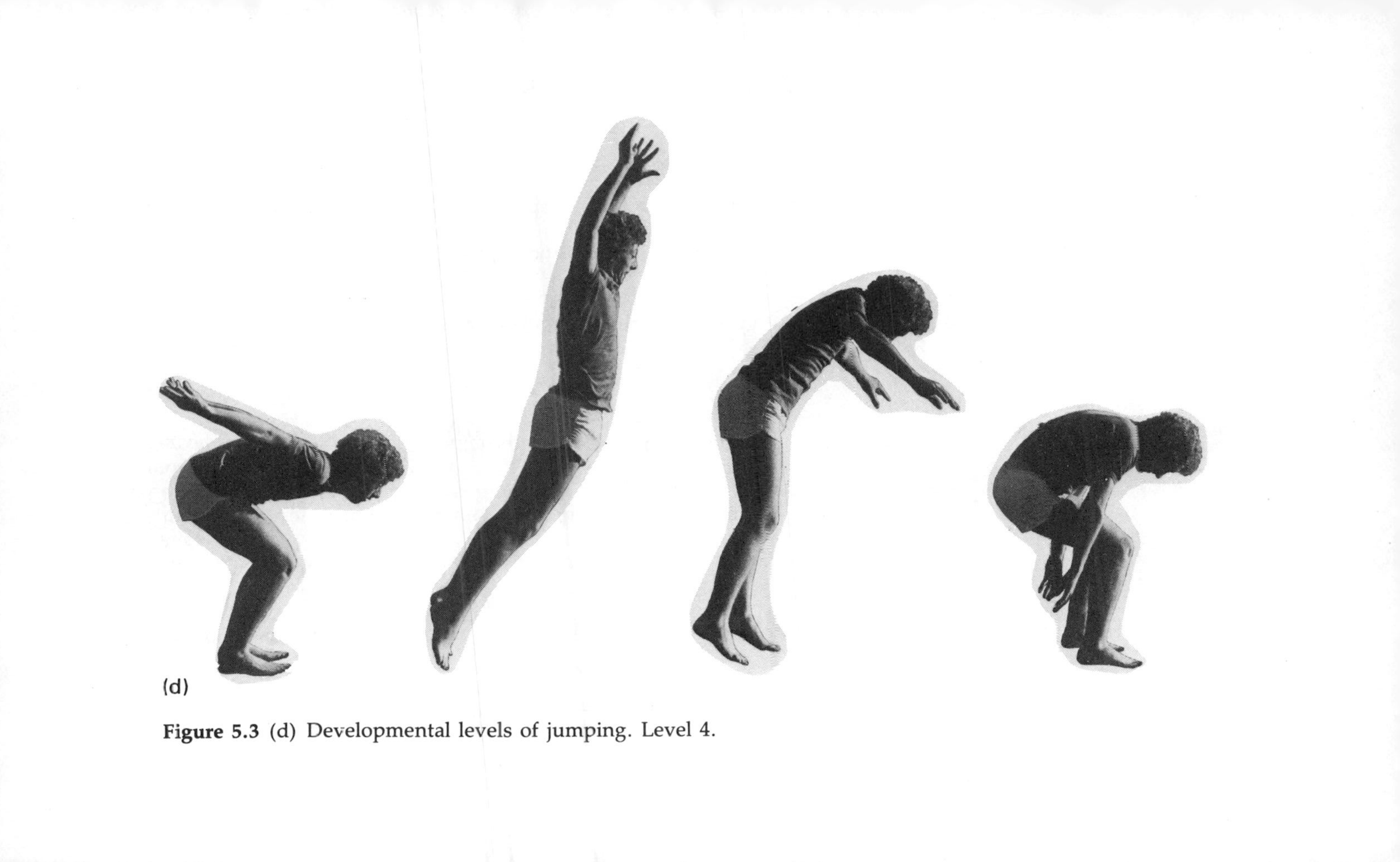

Figure 5.3 (d) Developmental levels of jumping. Level 4.

Table 5.4 Fundamental movement pattern for catching

CATCHING PROFILE

General body appearance

Level

1. Child faces thrower and performs stiff robot like action. Simultaneous upper limb movements: stiff arms and hands.
2. Child faces thrower in a stiff stance: uses total arm movement to catch ball.
3. Child faces thrower alert but less rigid than previous levels: greater use of arms and hands and some leg movements.
4. Person moves to a position to intercept the ball: uses upper and lower limbs effectively.

Upper body and limbs

Level

1. Hands and arms held at waist level ready to receive ball which is scooped in and trapped against the body.
2. Arms held forward and sideways at about waist level, fingers spread apart: ball clapped and caught away from body.
3. Arms usually held above waist level, elbows bent, hands together then parted to catch ball: ball clapped and caught away from body.
4. Moves with outstretched arms and hands to intercept balls moving in different directions and different speeds.

Lower body and limbs

Level

1. Lower limbs stiff, feet slightly apart and parallel: no change on catching the ball.

2. Feet parallel, some knee and hip movement as ball is caught.
3. Lower limbs used in catching action: final catching position is generally a semi-squat position.
4. Well coordinated movement of lower limbs to allow for different trajectory of balls: feet usually apart, one in front of the other.

Basis of movement pattern

Level

1. Ball is scooped in towards body once it touches part of the arm: no lower limb action: little range of joint movement.
2. Ball caught with clapping then scoop action: more total body and joint movement.
3. On catching the ball the arms are drawn towards the chest and the trunk is inclined forward: good joint movement.
4. As the ball is caught there is backward or sidewards movement of the arms and shoulders in line with flight of ball: good upper and lower limb coordination.

Additional criteria

Level

1. Apart from robot phase, there is no adjustment to the flight of the ball.
2. Characteristic avoidance response, of eyes shut/or head turned, as ball approaches the child.
3. Some upper and lower limb adjustments to changes in ball flight.
4. Complete body adjustment to different ball positions and ball flight.

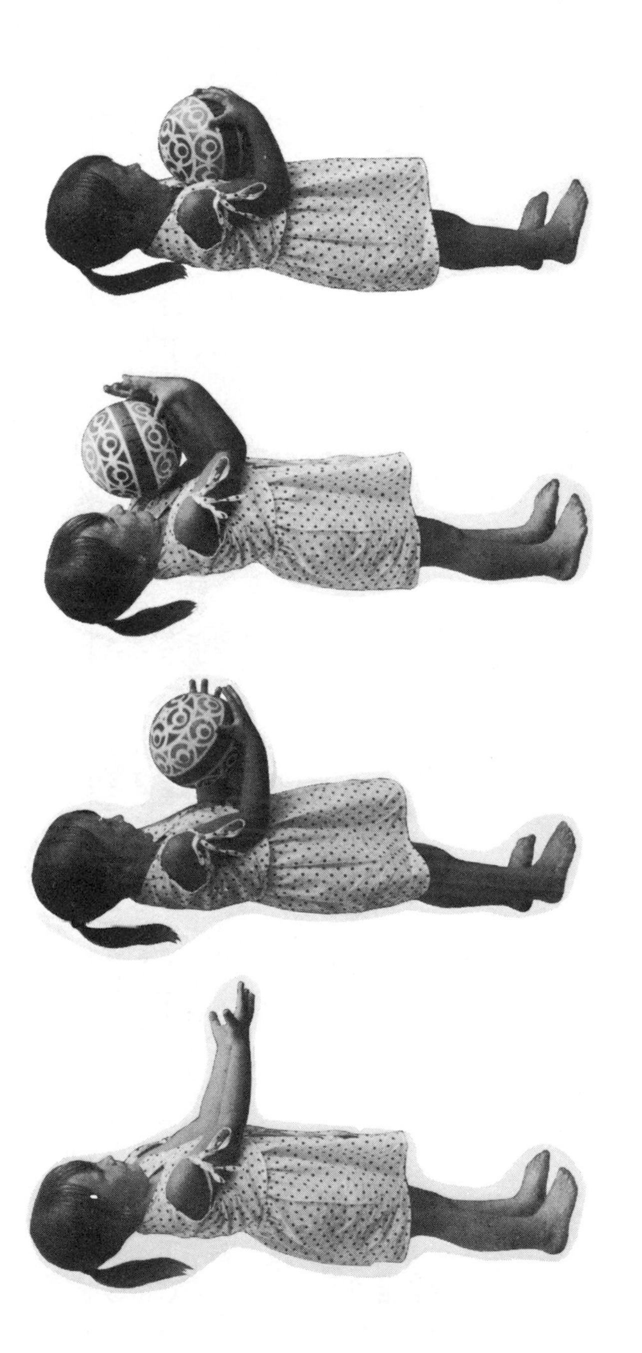

(a)

Figure 5.4 (a) Developmental levels of catching. Level 1.

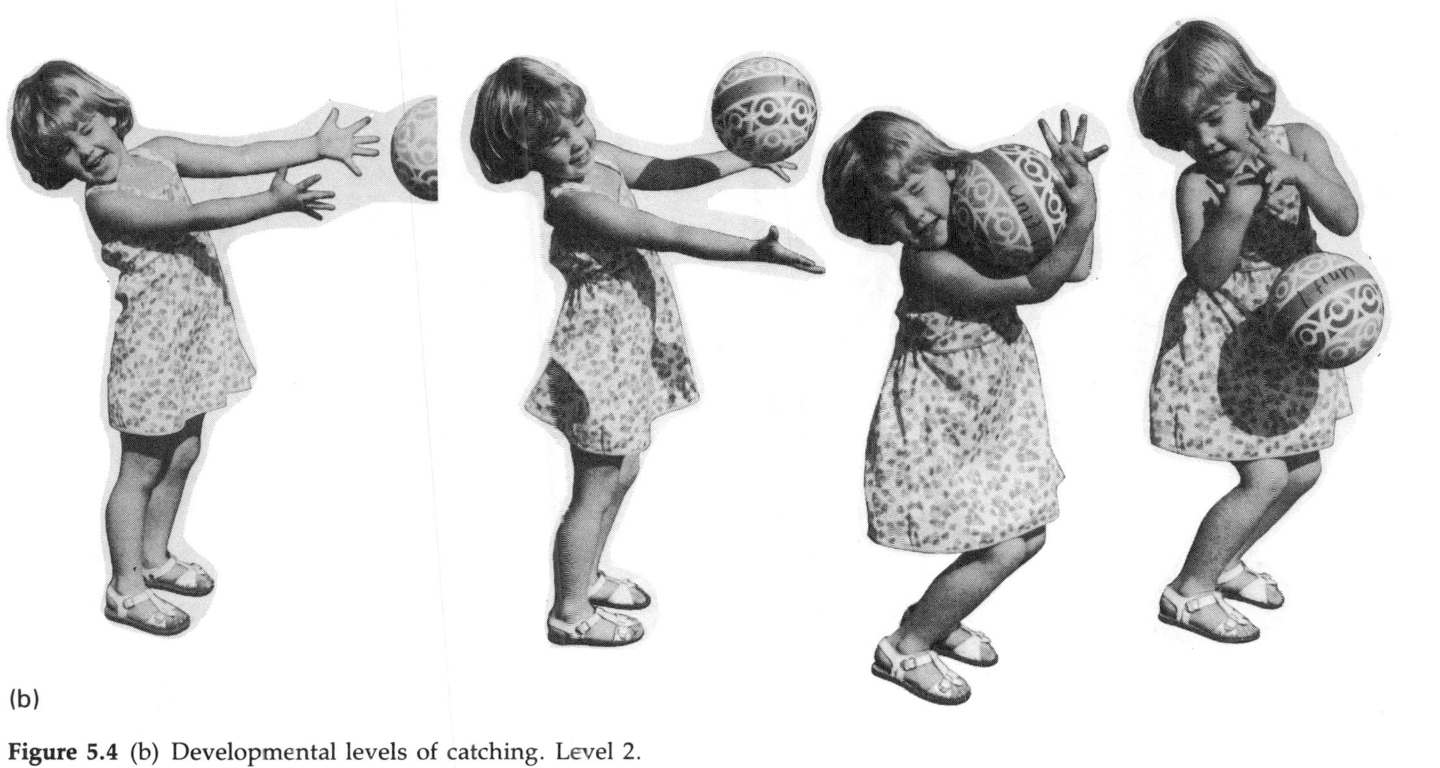

(b)

Figure 5.4 (b) Developmental levels of catching. Level 2.

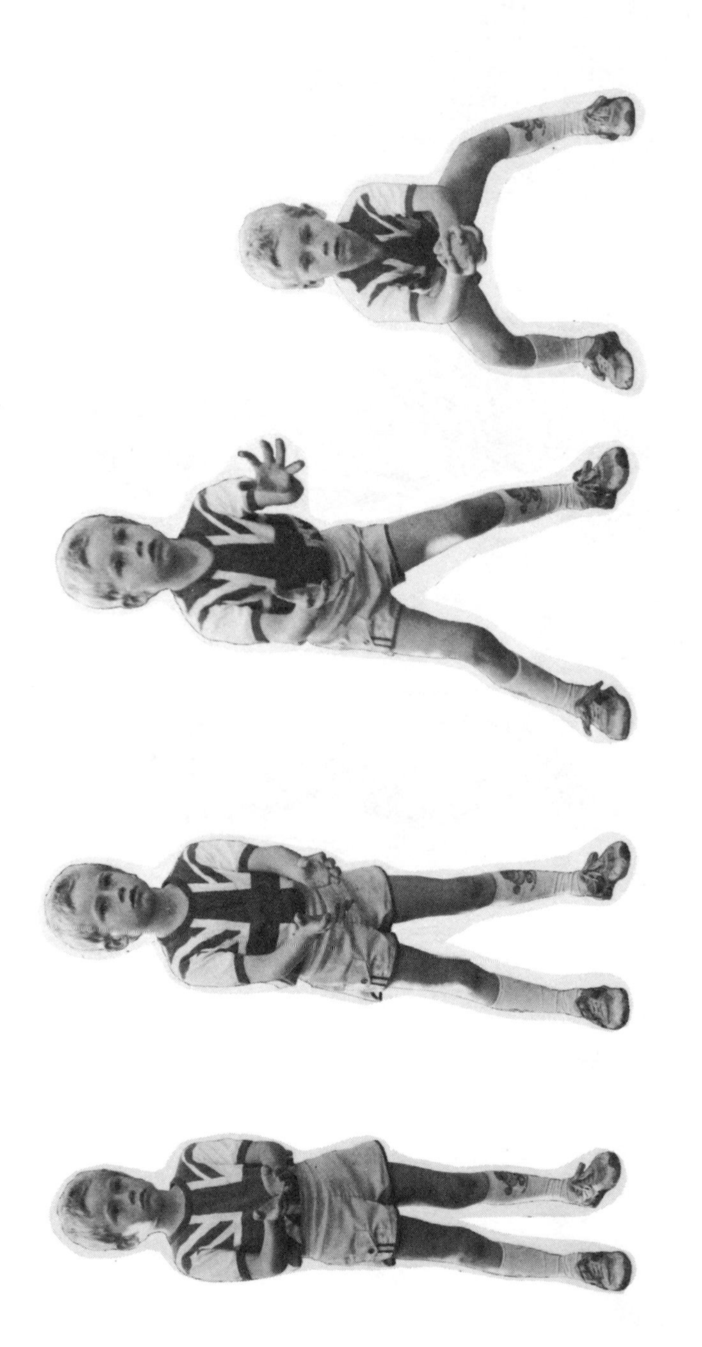

(c)

Figure 5.4 (c) Developmental levels of catching. Level 3.

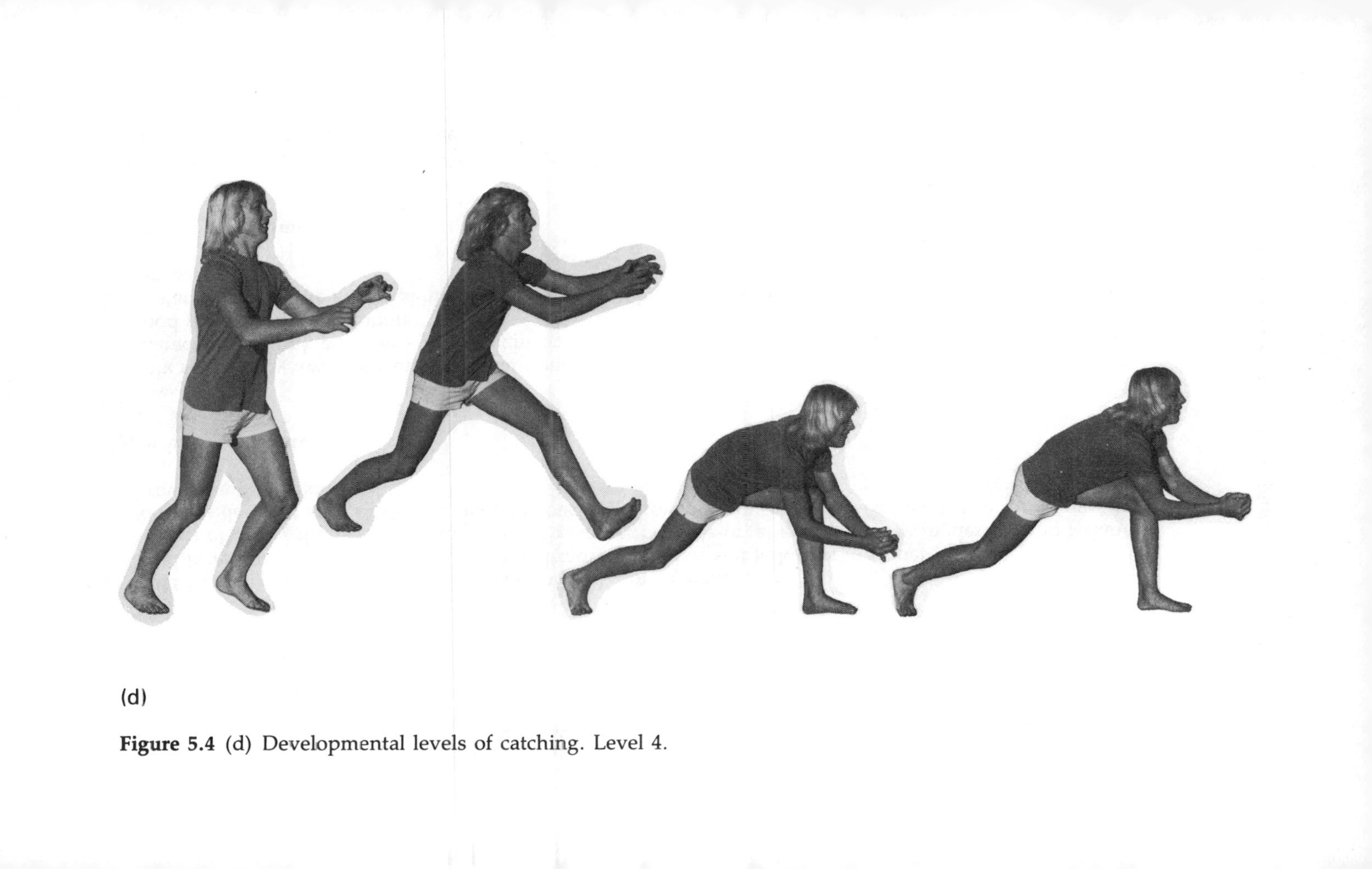

(d)

Figure 5.4 (d) Developmental levels of catching. Level 4.

Table 5.5 Fundamental movement pattern for throwing

THROWING PROFILE

General body appearance

Level

1. Child faces square on to target: uses stiff and jerky movements.
2. Child faces square on to target: coordinated movements but still jerkiness in upper limbs.
3. At start of throw the body is square on to the target but side-on at end of throw: moderate limb jerkiness.
4. Body is side-on at start of throw, same leg back as throwing arm: opposite leg forward to throwing arm at end of throw: smooth action.

Upper body and limbs

Level

1. Only slight body sway of trunk – forward and back simultaneously with arm action.
2. Characteristic trunk position – to the right on backswing – to the left on forward swing (right hand throw).
3. Good trunk and arm rotation.
4. At start of throw the arm is swung back with elbow bent at right angles: trunk rotates forward over front foot during throw.

Lower body and limbs

Level

1. Little or no leg movement: feet slightly apart and parallel to target.
2. Knee bent, no stepping action: feet parallel.

3. Characteristic step forward at start of throw on same side as throwing arm: feet together then apart.
4. Step forward with leg opposite to throwing arm: weight rocked back then forward.

Basis of movement pattern

Level

1. Throw dependent for force only on forward and backward movement of the throwing arm.
2. Force obtained form throwing arm together with trunk rotation.
3. Force obtained from arm swing and stepping action.
4. Force for throw obtained from effective use of both arms and legs as well as weight shift from back to front foot.

Additional criteria

Level

1. Very limited range of joint movement except in the throwing arm.
2. Greater use of upper body as well as the throwing arm.
3. Marked unilateral pattern of throwing arm and stepping foot.
4. Complete contralateral movement sequence of upper and lower limbs.

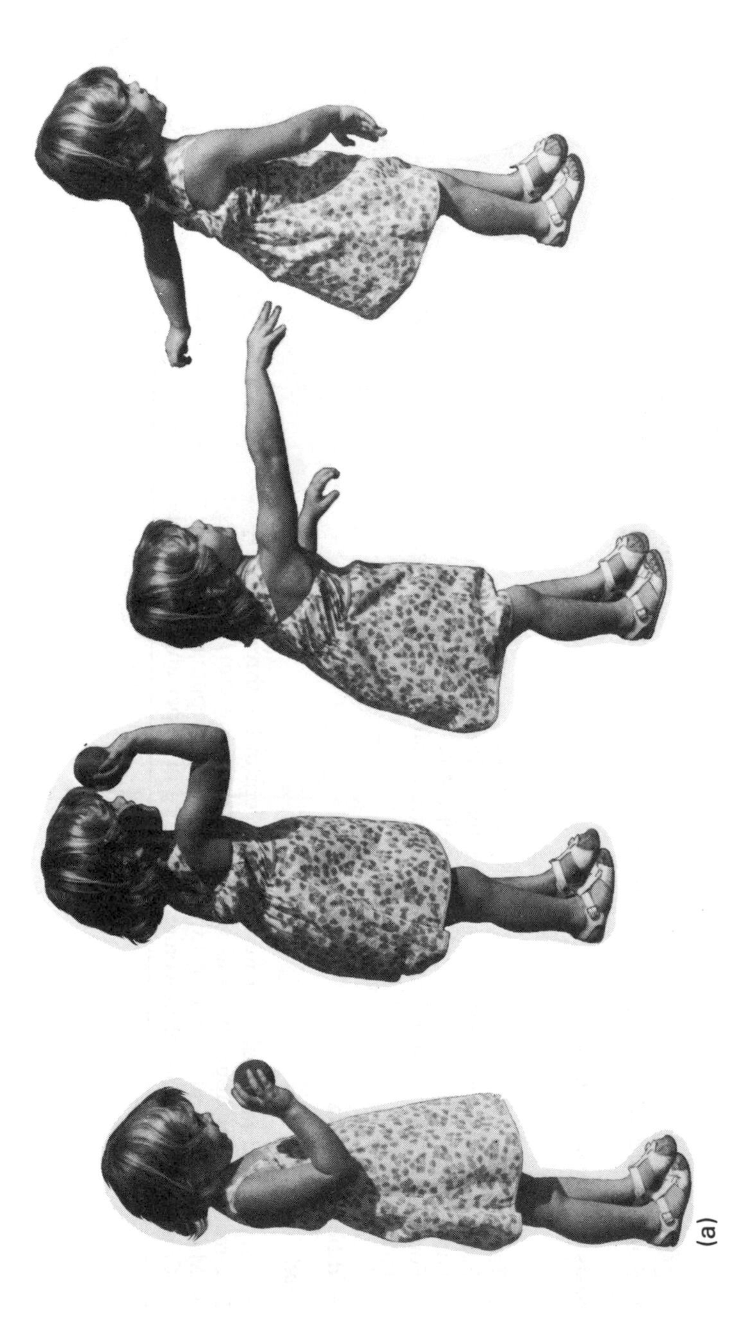

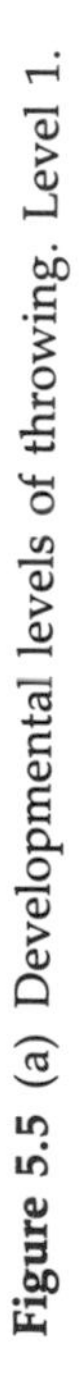

Figure 5.5 (a) Developmental levels of throwing. Level 1.

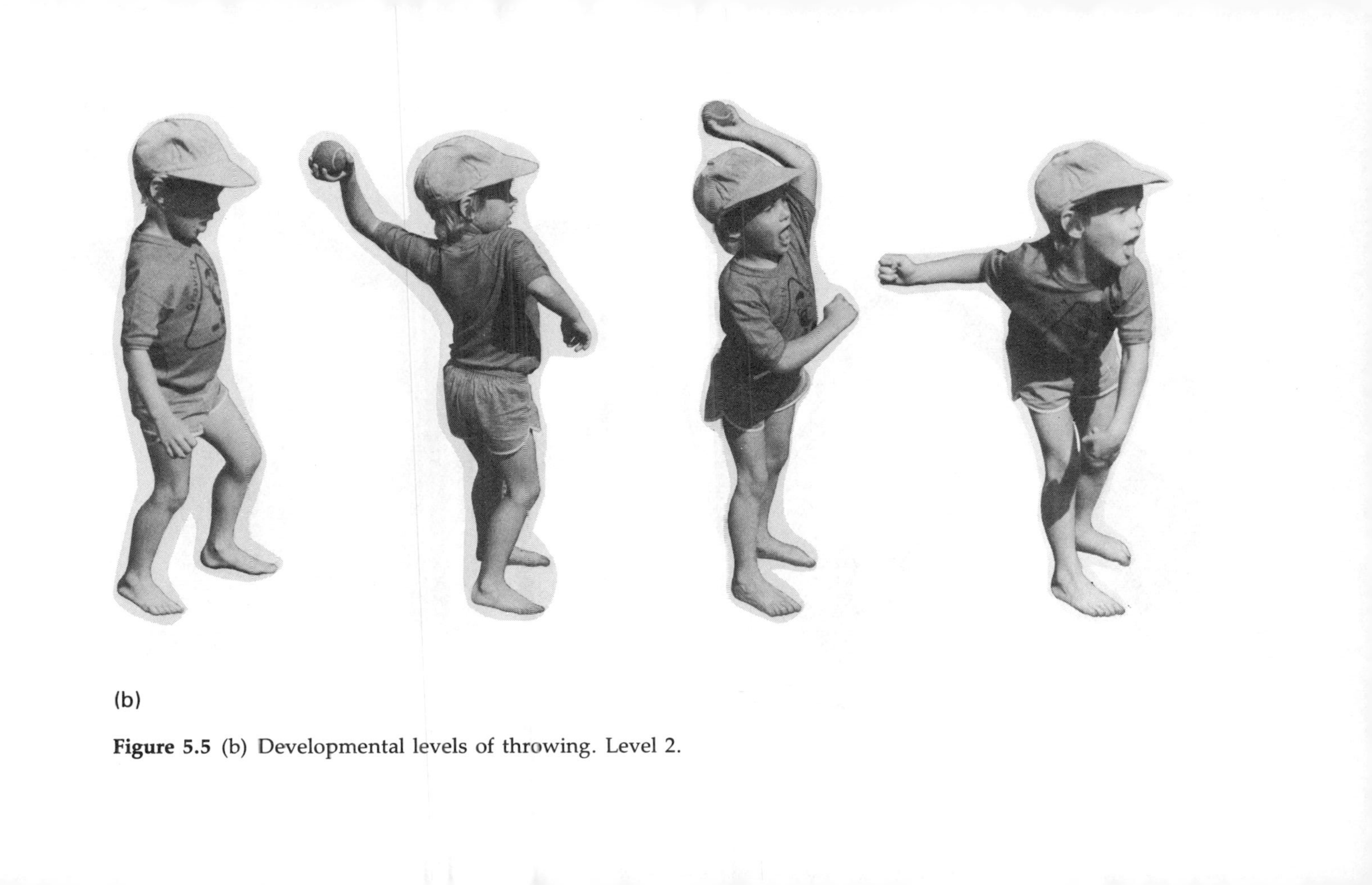

(b)

Figure 5.5 (b) Developmental levels of throwing. Level 2.

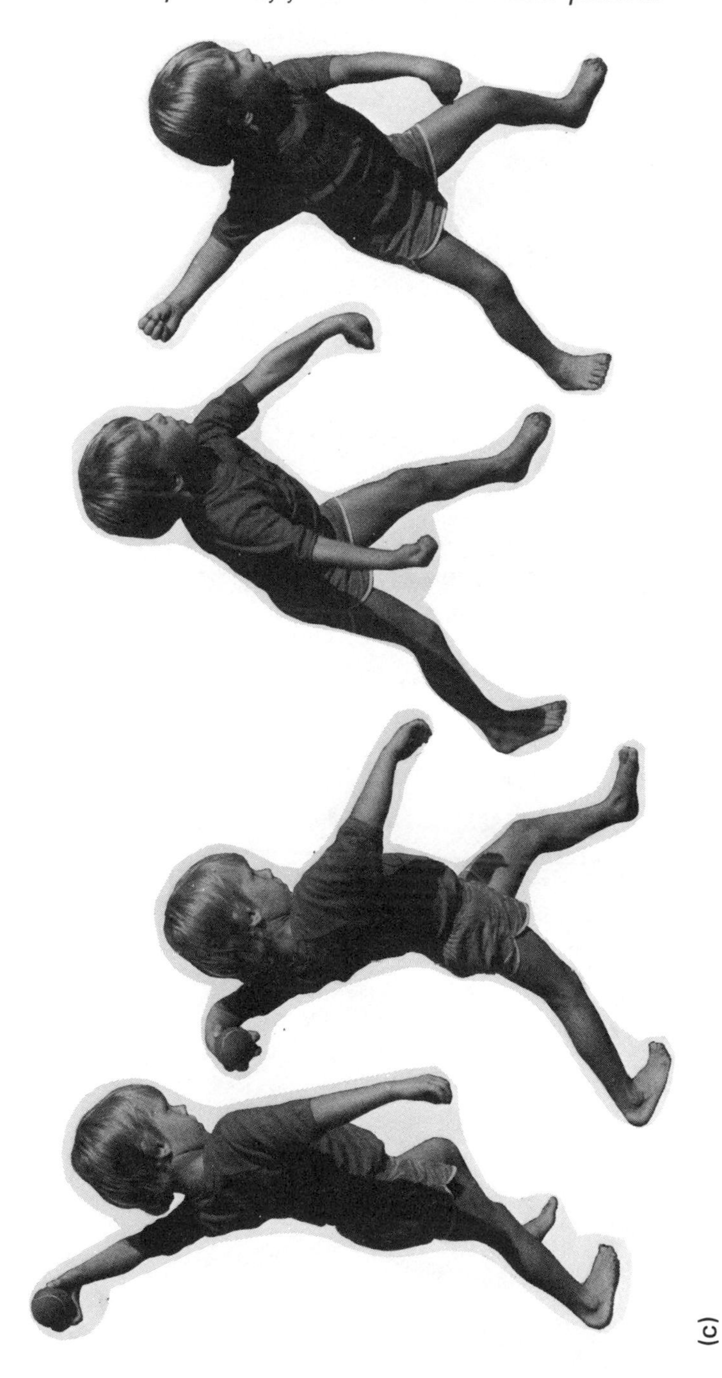

(c)

Figure 5.5 (c) Developmental levels of throwing. Level 3.

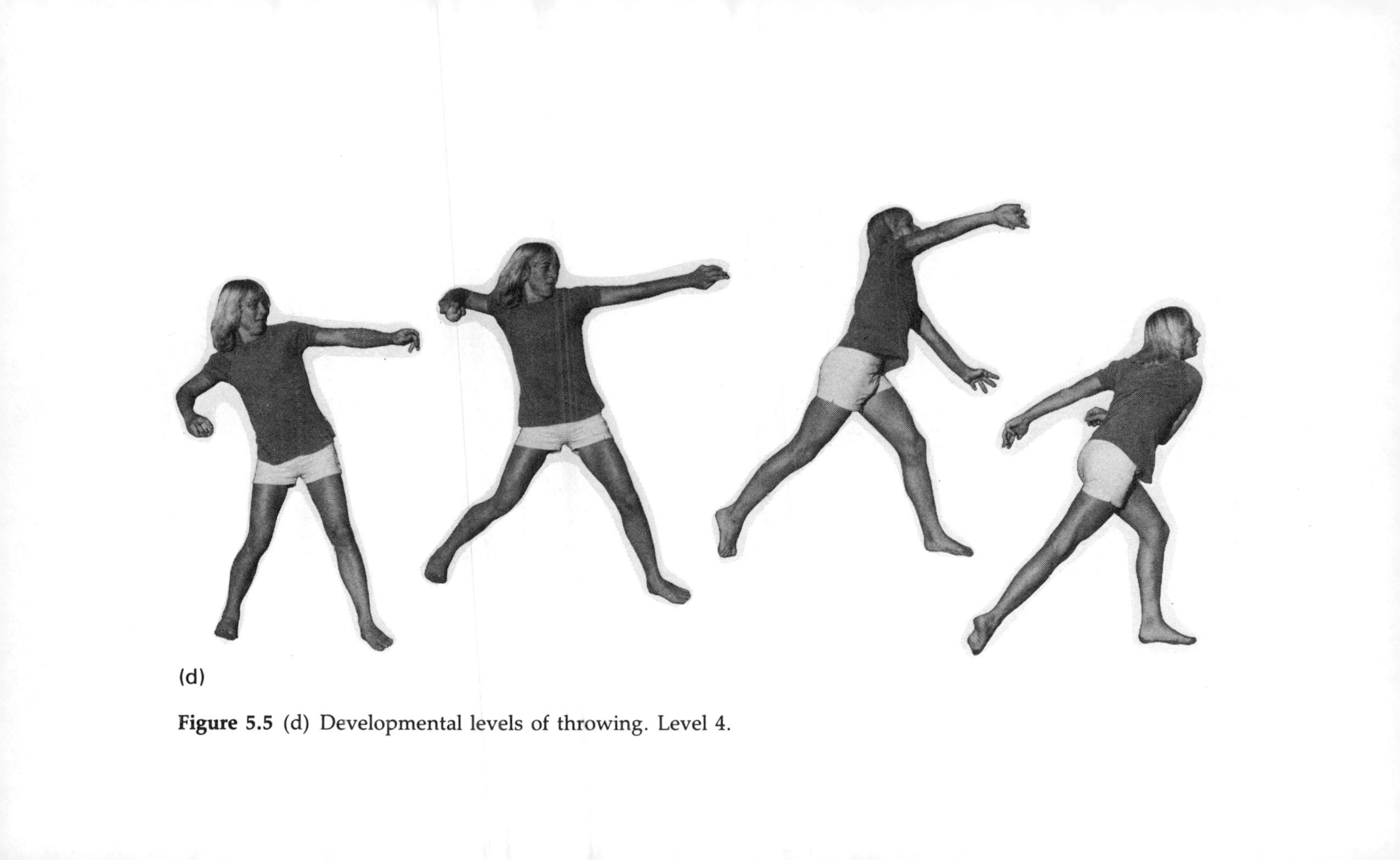

Figure 5.5 (d) Developmental levels of throwing. Level 4.

and 'lower body and limbs' divide the body into segments for easier observation of differences in children's fundamental movement patterns. 'General body appearance' presents an overall impression of the maturity of the movement profile, whereas the distinctive characteristic for each level of development within each movement is described in the section 'basis of the movement pattern'. The other more general element called 'additional criteria' was an attempt by the authors to determine changes in movement patterns which might be attributed to changes in underlying interlimb control, motor control, or control over the spatial–temporal aspects of the fundamental movement patterns.

The purpose of this study was to determine, first, whether the hypothesized sequences of development could be used to distinguish maturational and experiential changes in younger and older normally developing children. Second, to determine if the fundamental movement patterns could be used as instruments, not only to distinguish between movement pattern levels in younger (aged 4–7 years) and older (aged 8–12 years) children developing normally, but also in children who have been identified as having motor impairment.

DISCUSSION OF THE FUNDAMENTAL MOVEMENT PATTERN RESULTS

The results of the study (Appendix B gives more details of methodology and results) have demonstrated that the fundamental movement pattern check-lists differentiated among each of the groups studied. That is, of all the children who participated in the studies, the normally developing children were more mature than any of the other groups of children. Clumsy children were also more mature than the intellectually disabled and Down syndrome groups, respectively. An exception to this pattern of results was that normally developing and clumsy children did not differ significantly from one another in their total running pattern.

Results of the younger children

The younger normally developing children had more mature fundamental movement profiles than the intellectualy disabled and Down syndrome groups, whereas, there was a tendency in the jumping profile, and clear indication in throwing and catching, that children who are clumsy, intellectually disabled, or who have Down syndrome were at a similar level of maturity. The younger motor impaired children were about one level more mature in their locomotor patterns than in their manipulative patterns. Why this should be so is uncertain. There is, however, a similar but not so marked trend in normally developing children to have lower maturity in manipulative than locomotor patterns. It is possible that these results reflect less practice in throwing and catching patterns, than in the locomotor patterns.

Younger clumsy children were less mature than their normally developing peers in walking, whereas they were similar to the older intellectually disabled and Down syndrome groups in jumping. Moreover, younger clumsy children were less mature in throwing and catching than any of the these middle childhood groups, but they were more mature in this regard than the younger intellectually disabled and the younger Down syndrome groups. In fact, it would appear that throwing and catching profiles discriminate more between categories in the older than the younger children. It was also found that in the locomotor patterns of walking, running and jumping in younger children with intellectual disability and with Down syndrome were less mature than the other groups of children. Of interest, also, were the younger children with Down syndrome who were similar to intellectually disabled peers in walking, running, jumping and throwing, but lower in catching. Moreover, in all their patterns except catching, they were less mature than younger clumsy children.

Results of the older children

The results indicate that for the groups of children who were studied, the normally developing older children had attained quite mature levels in all of their movement patterns (walking, running, jumping, catching and throwing), but not the most mature level of these patterns. In contrast clumsy, intellectually disabled and Down syndrome children showed different patterns of development in terms of movement components, many of which were at a relatively immature level. For example, clumsy older children are more like normally developing younger children in terms of their walking, running and jumping profiles, but more advanced than the younger group in catching and throwing.

The older intellectually disabled children had acquired levels of movement patterns equivalent to younger normal children, and, older clumsy children in walking and running, but they were less mature in their jumping pattern than the younger normal children and the older clumsy children. In throwing and catching patterns they were similar to their age peers with Down syndrome, who in turn were more mature than children in early childhood, clumsy, intellectually disabled and Down syndrome children in throwing and catching actions.

Older children with Down syndrome had total walking patterns that were generally immature, in comparison with their clumsy and intellectually disabled peers. They were similar to intellectually disabled age peers in running, jumping, catching and throwing patterns, but were less mature than clumsy children of the same age in the same movement patterns.

General findings

Overall the results would suggest that observation of children's movement patterns, with the exception of throwing, enables the trained observer to discriminate well among younger and older groups of normally developing and clumsy children. The pattern of results, however, is less clear between older children with intellectual disability and Down syndrome and between younger clumsy, intellectually disabled and Down syndrome groups, particularly in the jumping, throwing and catching patterns.

Results for all the motor impaired children showed that they were delayed in the maturity of their movement patterns. An even more important finding was the apparently different pattern of progression through the movement patterns in children with Down syndrome, who were very immature in all fundamental movement patterns in early childhood but were closer to their intellectually disabled peers in middle childhood. Children with Down syndrome also showed considerable variation in the level of acquisition of their fundamental movement patterns, as they had less maturity in limb action in locomotor patterns and greater maturity in upper limb action than the intellectually disabled children.

CONCLUSIONS FROM THE STUDY

It is evident from these descriptions of qualitative changes, in the fundamental movement patterns of younger and older normally developing, clumsy intellectually disabled and children with Down syndrome, that the older group of children's movements are more complex. A possible developmental hierarchy is suggested by the data obtained from both age groups and in most of the movement patterns and elements of the movement patterns in normal and motor impaired children. There were significant differences, with the older groups at a more mature level than the younger age groups, in the five total movement profiles and in many of the elements which comprised the profiles used in this book. On the basis of these findings, it is claimed that the hypothesized movement profiles appear to describe sequences of movement which are based on developmental principles (Fischer and Farrar, 1988; Fischer and Lazerson, 1984).

The observational data reported here, however, do not support the claims made by early researchers (e.g. Hellebrandt *et al.*, 1961; Wild, 1938), that all children had acquired mature forms of the fundamental movement patterns by about 7 years of age. Nor does it support some of the more recent researchers, who are of the opinion that mature patterns are present at an early age, in walking (Sutherland *et al.*, 1980), running (Fortney, 1983), and jumping (Phillips, Clark and Petersen, 1985). Rather it appears that although some of the elements of a mature pattern may be present in young children who are motor impaired, they may not represent the most mature configuration of that pattern especially in terms of its spatial and temporal characteristics. Furthermore, it is possible that some of the observed elements of a movement pattern are based on synergies of movement which are present from an early age (see Chapter 6, for a discussion of units of movement called synergies), and, so do not really represent complex units of movement, but rather invariant characteristics of a movement pattern. In fact the results reported in this book, for the fundamental movement patterns are similar to the findings of Halverson, Roberton and Langendorfer (1982), who demonstrated that many of the mature configurations of the throwing pattern were still not present in 12 year old children even after extensive practice.

The findings in this study do not support Roberton's (1978) component model of fundamental movement profile progression. Roberton's theory was that components of movement patterns progress at a different rate from the total movement pattern (Halverson, Roberton and Langendorfer, 1982; Roberton, 1984). The model was derived from studies of the overarm throw, in which in one study (Roberton, 1978), little progress was noted in total patterns over a 2–3 year period. Nevertheless, she found more changes in the upper arm throwing component than in the lower body. An examination of the results (Appendix B) of the total scores in the throwing profile, do not support her contention of a different progression between the elements, as the level of maturity in each element comprising the throwing profile, in the data reported in this book, are similar.

Seefeldt's (1979; Seefeldt and Haubenstricker, 1982) contention, therefore, that children can be classified in terms of total body configuration is supported by the data reported in this book, especially in the movement element scores which were very similar to their total score for that movement profile. Moreover, the data showed that careful *in vivo* observation of children while they perform the fundamental movements (walking, running, jumping, catching and throwing), enables a person who is familiar with the profiles to ascertain different levels in maturity between total movement patterns and their components. It also enables the observer to distinguish between normal and clumsy children in early and middle childhood and in most cases between intellectually disabled and children with Down syndrome in the same age groups. Finally, it is suggested that the reported profiles should be used in a longitudinal study to verify whether children who are normal, clumsy, intellectually disabled or have Down syndrome actually do progress in a manner which has been observed in this cross-sectional study.

SUMMARY

The study on the fundamental movement profiles of two age groups of normally developing children, with and without motor impairment, and intellectually handicapped motor impaired children, would suggest that there is an age-related difference in the fundamental movement patterns of these children. This is because less mature levels were observed in the younger children and more mature levels in the older children, in all the fundamental movement patterns. Levels of maturity in the profiles and elements within the profiles, have also been shown to differ for each of the categories of motor impaired children. Thus, these results must cast some doubt on the hypothesis that motor impaired children are merely developmentally delayed.

Additionally, there is observational evidence that all the motor impaired children have less mature levels of motor control in terms of timing their movements, for instance, the jerkiness of younger intellectually disabled children and children with Down syndrome in their jumping and running actions. In particular, a neural synergy to control symmetry of lower limb movements appears deficient in younger children with Down syndrome. The theory of motor learning control is important to our understanding of the observed qualitative difference between normal and motor impaired children. A discussion of how motor control affects movement behaviour and the studies of motor control in normally developing and motor impaired children are found in Chapter 6.

REFERENCES

Ames, L.B. and Ilg, F.L. (1966) Individuality in motor development. *Journal of the American Physical Therapy Association*, **46**, 121–7.

Burnett, C.N. and Johnson, E.W. (1971a) Development of gait in childhood, Part 1: Method. *Developmental Medicine and Child Neurology*, **13**, 196–206.

Burnett, C.N. and Johnson, E.W. (1971b) Development of gait in childhood: Part 2. *Developmental Medicine and Child Neurology*, **13**, 207–15.

DiRocco, P.J., Clark, J.E. and Phillips, S.J. (1987) Jumping coordination patterns of mildly mentally retarded children. *Adapted Physical Activity Quarterly*, **4**, 178–91.

Dusenberry, L. (1952) A study of the effects of training in ball throwing by children ages three to seven. *Research Quarterly*, **23**, 9–14.

Fischer, K.W. and Farrar, M.J. (1988) Generalizations about generalizations: how a theory of skill development explains both generality and specificity, in *The Neo-Piagetian Theories of Cognitive Development: Towards an Integration*, (ed. A. Demetriou), North-Holland, Elsevier, Amsterdam, pp. 137–71.

Fischer, K.W. and Lazerson, A. (1984) *Human Development*. W.H. Freeman, New York.

Fortney, V.L. (1983) The kinematics and kinetics of the running pattern of two-, four- and six-year-old children. *Research Quarterly for Exercise and Sport*, **54**, 126–35.

Gesell, A. (1973) *The First Five Years of Life*. Methuen, London.

Halverson, L.E., Roberton, M.A. and Langendorfer, S. (1982) Development of the overarm throw: movement and ball velocity changes by seventh grade. *Research Quarterly for Exercise and Sport*, **53**, 198–205.

Hellebrandt, F.A., Rarick, L., Glassow, R. and Carns, M.L. (1961) Physiological analysis of basic motor skills: 1. Growth and development of jumping. *American Journal of Physical Medicine*, **40**, 14–25.

Hicks, J.A. (1930) The acquisition of motor skills in young children: a study of the effects of practice in throwing at a moving target. *Child Development*, **1**, 90–105.

O'Brien, C.C. (1994) Motor development and learning in children, in *The Early Years* (eds G. Boulton-Lewis and D. Catherwood), The Australian Council for Educational Research, Victoria, Australia, pp. 145–85.

O'Brien, C.C. (1988) *Motor development in clumsy, intellectually disabled and Down's syndrome children: A Comparative Study*. Unpublished PhD thesis, University of Queensland.

O'Brien, C.C. and Hayes, A. (1989) Motor development in early childhood of clumsy, intellectually disabled and Down's Syndrome children. *ACHPER National Journal*, **124**, 15–19.

Parker, A.W. and Bronks, R. (1980) Gait of children with Down's Syndrome. *Archives of Physical Medicine and Rehabilitation*, **61**, 345–51.

Parker, A.W., Bronks, R. and Snyder, C.W. (1986) Walking patterns in Down's Syndrome. *Journal of Mental Deficiency Research*, **30**, 317–30.

Phillips, S.J., Clark, J.E. and Petersen, R.D. (1985) Developmental differences in standing long jump takeoff parameters. *Journal of Human Movement Studies*, **11**, 75–87.

Roberton, M.A. (1977a) Stability of stage categorizations across trials: implications for the 'Stage Theory' of overarm throw development. *Journal of Human Movement Studies*, **3**, 49–59.

Roberton, M.A. (1977b) Stability of stage categorizations in motor development, in *Psychology of Motor Behavior and Sport*, (eds D.M. Landers and R.W. Christina), Human Kinetics, Champaign, IL, pp. 494–506.

Roberton, M.A. (1978) Longitudinal evidence for developmental stages in the forceful overarm throw. *Journal of Human Movement Studies*, **4**, 167–75.

Roberton, M.A. (1984) Changing motor patterns during childhood, in *Motor Development During Childhood and Adolescence*, (ed. J.R. Thomas), Burgess, Minneapolis, pp. 48–90.

Roberton, M.A. and Di Rocco, P. (1981) Validating a motor skill sequence for mentally retarded children. *American Corrective Therapy Journal*, **35**, 148–54.

Roberton, M.A., Williams, K. and Langendorfer, S. (1980) Prelongitudinal screening of motor developmental sequences. *Research Quarterly for Exercise and Sport*, **51**, 724–31.

Seefeldt, V. (1979) Developmental motor patterns: implications for elementary school physical education, in *Psychology of Motor Behavior and Sport* (eds C.H. Nadeau, W.R. Halliwell, K.M. Newell, and G.C. Roberts), Human Kinetics, Champaign, IL, pp. 314–23.

Seefeldt, V. and Haubenstricker, J. (1982) Patterns, phases or stages: an analytical model for the study of developmental movement, in *The Development of Movement Control and Co-ordination*, (eds J.A.S. Kelso and J.E. Clark), John Wiley, Chichester, pp. 309–18.

Shirley, M.M. (1931) *The First Two Years*. University of Minnesota Press, Minneapolis.

Sinclair, C.B. (1973) *Movement of the Young Child: Ages Two to Six*. Charles E. Merrill, Columbus, OH.

Sutherland, D.H., Olsen, R., Cooper, L. and Woo, S.L.Y. (1980) The development of mature gait. *Journal of Bone and Joint Surgery*, **62A**, 336–53.

Wellman, B.L. (1937) Motor achievement of preschool children. *Childhood Education*, **13**, 311–16.

Wheelwright, E.F., Minns, R.A., Elton, R.A. and Law, H.T. (1993) Temporal and spatial parameters of gait in children, II:

Pathological gait. *Developmental Medicine and Child Neurology*, **35**, 114–25.

Wild, M.R. (1938) The behavior pattern of throwing and some observations concerning its course of development in children. *Research Quarterly*, **9**, 20–4.

6

Motor control

The aim of this chapter is to examine relevant literature and experimental evidence to ascertain whether there are any differences in motor control processes between normally developing and motor impaired children. Motor control is the third aspect of movement behaviour examined in this book, in order to gain a more comprehensive basis for assessing and understanding the development of children with motor impairment. Motor control theory is important because it provides a conceptual framework for examining movement behaviour, particularly skilled movements. This chapter also reports results from the experimental interlimb bimanual task which was chosen to determine advanced processes in children's movement behaviour. Interlimb bimanual coordination is an integral part of many complex movements used in everyday tasks, sports, recreation, leisure, school and work.

OVERVIEW

Skilled voluntary movement is defined by behavioural scientists, as the most efficient action to achieve a specific movement. A skilled movement appears fluent because it successfully meets the spatial and temporal requirements inherent in the task (Keogh and Sugden, 1985; Sparrow, 1983). It is suggested that less-efficient motor control and response organization in young children is partly why there is an observable difference between the movement behaviour of young children and adults, as has been argued in the preceding chapters (see also, Charlton, 1992; Clark, 1982; Fagard, 1987).

Further, it is suggested, therefore, that in order to gain a more comprehensive understanding of movement skill development in children, it is important to study the changes which occur in underlying control processes as the child becomes more competent at achieving movement goals (Connolly, 1986; Smyth, 1986).

Early motor control studies did not really help us in this regard because they concentrated on how adults organized motor responses for highly skilled movements such as those used in handwriting and typing (e.g. Viviani and Terlzuolo, 1980). More recently, however, interest has been shown in children's bimanual control of the upper limbs (Fagard, 1987) and the phasing of interlimb control of the lower limbs in locomotor patterns (Clark and Whitall, 1989; Roberton and Halverson, 1989).

The reason, then, for studying processes underlying motor skill development is to gain an holistic perspective of some of the changes that occur in movement behaviour as children develop (Gallagher and Thomas 1986; Mounoud, 1986). Such an approach to understanding motor skill development extends the more traditional description of changes that have already been examined in this book, in movement patterns such as running or jumping. Instead, it attempts to define the changes in the underlying control processes which contribute to these differences. This chapter then seeks to understand the developmental progression in skilled movements, in relation to how complex movement patterns are controlled by the central nervous system. Some of the theorists who have sought to provide an explanation of motor control will be discussed in the next section.

Motor learning and control theories

As was discussed in Chapter 1 (pp. 15–20) these theories can be divided into divergent approaches. These are: (1) those that view motor learning and control as reliant on central representation of movement; (2) those that view motor control as occurring without the necessity for central representation of movement; and (3) an attempt to integrate these two approaches in what is known as the ecological psychological approach to motor learning and control.

Despite different theories adopted by motor learning and control theorists, they have all sought an understanding of the processes that control groups of muscles in a coordinated fashion, once a response has been selected. In other words they are seeking the theoretical framework which delineates 'the language of movements' (Stelmach and Diggles, 1982, p. 83). An ecological psychological approach to motor control has been adopted, by the authors, as this approach appears to best explain the holistic concept of coordination processes adopted in this book (Whiting, Vogt and Vereijken, 1992).

As mentioned in Chapter 1, one of the early researchers who influenced the study of motor control was Bernstein (1967), who stated that in understanding motor coordination it is necessary to explain how the body controls the large number of joints that make up a coordinated movement. He was of the opinion that the only way to control such a large number of variables was by a system of constraints. Such constraints have been called synergies by later researchers (Craske and Craske, 1986; Hinton, 1984; Lee, 1984).

Another notion of Bernstein (1967), and later researchers (Arbib, 1984; Glencross, 1980), was that complex movements are controlled by a hierarchical system. There is a general consensus that voluntary control of movement, in hierarchical control models, requires some sort of intention or preplanning (termed action plan, or a generalized motor programme) before initiation of the movement (Arbib, 1980; Glencross, 1980; Newell, 1980; Schmidt, 1988). The problem with these theories is that it is difficult to find any empirical evidence to support them. Nevertheless, these theories are conceptually important and will be discussed in the next section.

It is not difficult, however, to measure the less abstract manifestations of motor control, such as timing and force of movements (Ivry, 1986; Keele, Ivry and Pokorny, 1987), which can be observed in adults and children who are relatively skilled in motor performance and who have apparently fluent fundamental movement patterns. These aspects of motor control, from an ecological perspective, will also be discussed in the next section.

Hierarchical and multilevel motor control

Hierarchical motor control is divided into single or multilevel control depending upon the number of levels of transformation that occur before movement signals reach the muscles. An example of single level motor control is the early notion of a motor programme proposed by Keele (1981). In this early conceptualization, a motor programme was a set of centrally stored commands that specified all the parameters of the desired movement. This conceptualization of control was later refuted, mainly because other researchers considered that it would place an unrealistic load on the central command system. Another objection to the notion of a motor programme was that it would not allow any flexibility in an ongoing movement, because more peripheral areas of the body would be harder to control because they are dependent on signals from the central command system (Stelmach and Diggles, 1982). In contrast to the notion of hierarchical control, multilevel control acknowledges that many patterns of movement are initiated at the spinal cord level, thus allowing for greater flexibility in movement control. One of the models that places a great deal of emphasis on horizontal transference of information in the central nervous system is the one proposed by Arbib (1980, 1984). This model suggests that a number of schemas interact to achieve a desired movement.

A general consensus in the literature, is that there is some sort of intention or preplanning of a movement. This notion has resulted in a number of theories on how this occurs and a range of terms to describe the key processes (Colley and Beech, 1988). For instance, central control has been called an action plan (Newell, 1980), a recall schema (Schmidt, 1980, 1988) and interacting schemas (Arbib, 1980, 1984). According to other theorists generation of the action plan relies on feedforward (Arbib, 1984; Bernstein, 1967), that is, there is an interaction of task and environmental factors prior to setting the parameters for the desired movement. This process is then followed by the central nervous system generating the signals which will control the muscles used in the movement. It should be noted that all these theorists have attempted to explain how the initial control processes are formulated but they have differed in the details of how these executive or overall control systems would operate.

A widely held concept on how the central nervous system might control movement once the action plan is formulated, was proposed by Schmidt (1980, 1988), who claimed that there is a generalized motor programme for any one class of skills. These generalized programmes are assumed to contain the prestructured commands for many movements, which together with specific response specifications are incorporated in the final stages of the programme. This would mean that a generalized motor programme for throwing a ball could be modified by specific parameter instructions, for example, to speed up or slow down the movement sequence before it begins (Schmidt 1980).

It is claimed that a generalized motor programme has some similarities with the ideas of Bernstein (Arbib, 1984) because it can also be incorporated with Schmidt's schema theory (Schmidt, 1988). For example, Schmidt's theory has two parts, a recall schema, which has a function similar to Bernstein's notion of feedforward, and a response schema, which is similar to his notion of feedback. In schema theory, feedforward can be thought of as an anticipatory mechanism which integrates the person's motor control system with environmental factors, while feedback supplies the motor control system with information about errors to enable corrections to be made in subsequent movements (Newell, Morris and Scully, 1985).

Schema theory also accommodates the concept of muscle synergies that are incorporated in many movements, for instance in postural stabilization; cyclic locomotor synergies for walking, running and swimming and synergies for throwing, striking and jumping (Arbib, 1984). A broad concept of synergies or schemas has been outlined which claims that movement is dependent upon a system of interacting schemas. As an example, the simple act of walking down the street involves the interaction of synergies or schemas for 'walking (including maintaining posture); breathing, talking, gesticulating; and scanning the shop windows' (Arbib, 1984, pp. 551–552.) Thus, internal movement commands are also dependent on environmental information if a movement goal is to be achieved. Similar theorizing that the environment is as important as the motor command system is found in other holistic notions of motor control (Reed, 1982; Turvey and Kugler, 1984; Turvey, Shaw and Mace, 1978).

Synergies, or other names for them such as muscle linkages or units of action, appear to be the intermediate level of control in the movement hierarchy. That is, they represent a processing stage between action plans and individual muscle contractions. Evidence for the existence of synergies has been provided by locomotor studies (e.g. Clark and Whitall, 1989; Deitz, 1992; Patla, 1985; Roberton and Halverson, 1988; Shapiro *et al.*, 1981; Shik and Orlovsky, 1976; Winter, 1983). It is also feasible that synergies may evolve from well-learnt movement patterns, where the muscular force and the rhythm of the movement are so automated that the muscle linkages form part of the subsystem of the movement (Lee, 1984). The major advantage of an intermediate level of motor control, such as one at the level of muscle synergies, is that it reduces the attentional load when performing a complex movement because groups of muscles can be activated as a unit, rather than individually (Stelmach and Diggles, 1982).

Control of complex movements

How the body copes with complex movements in terms of the rhythmic and spatial parameters, is still the subject of much research. According to action theorists, rhythmic control of movement is based on the idea that muscle linkages can operate like oscillators to produce an ongoing rhythmical response (Craske and Craske, 1986; Greene, 1982). Such an approach was adopted to research the production of handwriting, in which it was claimed that coupled oscillators, one moving in a horizontal and one in a vertical direction would produce conventional script. More recent evidence suggests that sequences of complex movements may be produced by phases of oscillations between sets of muscles or some form of linkage between the limbs used to perform the task (Swinnen and Walter, 1991).

Another concept in relation to the production of accurate spatial–temporal components of a movement is that of tuning. Tuning refers to the transformation of abstract representations of movement into specific muscle actions. It is believed that tuning is accomplished through feedforward and feedback mechanisms to the central nervous system. Lower motor control centres, however, such as the spinal generators also appear to be involved in the tuning process especially in relation to temporal characteristics of the movement (Deitz, 1992). Even though it has been shown that movement synergies can be controlled from the spinal cord level, the predetermined aspects of such movements would not be able to be modified because they are reflex in nature (Keele, 1981; Schmidt, 1980; Summers, 1975; Viviani and Terzuolo, 1980). It has been claimed that components of movements that cannot be easily modified are produced automatically, (i.e. these aspects are known as invariant components of a movement). Invariant components of complex movements have been identified in the walking, runnning, hopping, galloping and skipping patterns. In these locomotor patterns the relative phasing of the limbs in each lower limb cycle has been shown to remain constant despite differences in the speed of the action, or the maturity of the action (Clark and Whitall, 1989; Ferrandez and Pailhouse, 1986; Roberton and Halverson, 1988; Shapiro *et al.*, 1981). Other movement parameters, many of which are affected more by peripheral factors such as visual information, enable variations to be made to a movement while it is in progress and so allow for more flexibility in movement behaviour.

The type of hypothetical motor control which has been described in this section is more in keeping with current theories and research, in that voluntary control of movement has shifted from studies of input and output processes, to the examination of recent theories related to the control of movement (Abernathy and Sparrow, 1992). The need for such a shift in emphasis was expressed by Whiting (e.g. Whiting, Vogt and Vereijken, 1992) who argued that in order to understand control processes in real-life situations it is necessary to study skills which require more complex control than previous experiments which more frequently studied simple laboratory tasks.

It is mainly for this reason that an interlimb coordination task was chosen as an experimental topic for research on motor control in normally developing and motor impaired children. In addition, interlimb coordination was considered pertinent because changes in upper and lower limb occur at different levels of the fundamental movement patterns, as well as in highly skilled movements. Before reporting the study it is pertinent to review studies relevant to general motor control in both groups of children.

MOTOR CONTROL STUDIES IN CHILDREN

Some experiments have investigated motor control tasks, other than bimanual tasks. These tasks generally have shown that children under 10 years of age cannot control the parameters of a movement as well as adults (e.g. Burton, 1986, 1987; Guiard, 1987). Nevertheless, it should be noted that the difference in ability among younger and older children and adults may not only be related to ability to control parameters of a movement but also may be due to differences in ability to develop adequate cognitive strategies to encode and reproduce movements (Gallagher and Thomas, 1986).

The earlier motor control studies on children have mainly concentrated on single limb movements or discrete actions. Schellekens, Kalverboer and Scholten (1984), for instance, found that when they tested children on a reciprocal tapping task, that was either self or task paced, movement time decreased with increased age. Burton (1986) found an age-related improvement in internal timing consistency in repetitive movements and a decrease in the time to organize a complex response.

Perhaps more ecologically valid evidence of motor control processes can be found in the changes in limb coordination and timing in fundamental locomotor patterns. The progressive development of these locomotor patterns seems to indicate there is an age-related improvement in the manner in which children control complex movement patterns (Brown and Parker, 1992; Ferrandez and Pailhouse, 1986; Roberton and Halverson, 1988). Furthermore, the literature review and studies in this book which addressed fundamental movement patterns, indicated that motor control improvement is age-related, because of the observed changes in phasing between alternating limb movements and the symmetry of the action. Similarly, the same inferences could be made for children who are clumsy, intellectually disabled, or have Down syndrome, who exhibit delayed and different development, resulting in movement patterns different from those of normally developing children (O'Brien, 1988).

Clumsy and intellectually disabled children are portrayed as slower, less coordinated and more variable in their motor behaviour than normal children (Smyth, 1991, 1992), so it seems that they may have underlying problems with coordination and control of movement (Hoover and Wade, 1985). These problems in coordination, however, have not been widely researched in intellectually disabled children or clumsy children by a motor control paradigm incorporating complex movements. This has meant that most of the evidence of deficits in motor control come from research on children and young adults with Down syndrome on relatively simple movement tasks. These studies will now be reviewed.

Motor control studies on children with Down syndrome

Frith and Frith (1974) sought underlying components which would account for observed clumsiness in children with Down syndrome. In order not to confuse task performance with disability, children were matched for performance on a pursuit tracking task and Frostig's test of visual perception. This matching procedure resulted in quite large chronological age differences between the groups, as the mean ages were 17 years for the children with Down syndrome, 12 years for autistic children and nearly 6 years for the normal control group. All the children were tested on a rotary pursuit tracking task (which was too difficult for most subjects) and a tapping task. In the tapping task the children were required to tap as fast as possible using the same finger on a 13 x 7 cm panel for 90 seconds.

These researchers found that as a group children with Down syndrome were slower at tapping, and, unlike the other groups they also failed to improve on the rotary pursuit task. On the basis of these findings, Frith and Frith (1974) suggested that such children are unable to formulate an adequate motor programme to control a relatively simple motor task such as a sequence of taps. Furthermore, they suggested that much of the observed slowness in movement in this group can be attributed to the necessity for these children to rely heavily on sensory feedback to perform the movement, which is a very slow method of control.

Hogg and Moss (1983) also observed very slow movements in children with Down syndrome (aged 44 months), in comparison with normal children (aged 36 months). They found that their movements were slow even though the matching task (based on rod size and orientation) had no time constraints. Once again the slowness of movements in children with Down syndrome appears to be indicative of delays in processing, and response selection of movement parameters, both of which are underlying motor control factors.

Seyfort and Spreen (1979) attempted to determine if children with Down syndrome really do have problems in formulating motor programmes for predetermined sequences of movement by using a different tapping task from the one used by Frith and Frith (1974). They compared 18 people with Down syndrome (aged 12–30 years) with intellectually disabled people of similar age and IQ scores (between 36 and 55). Their task involved a tapping sequence between two plates (2.2 cm in diameter and 3.3 cm apart) for a 60 seconds time period. The results revealed no difference in tapping rate between the two groups. Nevertheless, the fact that the Down syndrome group made significantly more errors, by not tapping alternately, once again supports the notion that they may have a deficit in formulating a motor programme.

In a review of simple and choice reaction time experiments it has been reported that children with Down syndrome of the same chronological age as intellectually disabled children have a slower premotor reaction time (Henderson, 1985). The finding that children with Down syndrome have a slower reaction time than other groups of children, however, may not necessarily apply to complex movement tasks (Hoover and Wade, 1985). This is because simple and choice reaction experimental tasks generally are in response to an auditory or visual stimulus, so the movement cannot be preplanned and the actual movements are over a short distance. Such tasks, therefore, do not appear to have sufficient ecological validity to predict performance in more complex everyday situations.

Davis and Kelso (1982) addressed the problem of hypotonia in an attempt to find underlying problems in muscle control and coordination in individuals aged between 14 and 21 years who had Down syndrome and whose IQ scores were in the range from 25–60. Hypotonia is a characteristic of persons with Down syndrome that may make it difficult for them to set muscular stiffness parameters around joint angles. Their results indicated that persons with Down syndrome, when compared with normal individuals, are similar in their ability to specify resting muscular length–tension parameters, but they apparently were unable voluntarily to increase muscular stiffness.

In order to extend the findings from this earlier study, Davis and Sinning (1987) tried to determine whether muscular stiffness can be changed in normal, intellectually disabled and adult males with Down syndrome, by a weight training programme. The training consisted of exercise for elbow flexion for three sessions a week for 8 weeks. These training sessions appeared to have little effect on the ability to set muscular stiffness in all the groups who participated. The results also showed that people with Down syndrome were only able to generate a small amount of muscular force and were less able to maintain a constant muscular force against resistance than normal and intellectually disabled people. According to these authors, their results confirm that people with Down syndrome have an underlying motor control problem, in that they appear unable voluntarily to control muscular stiffness for movement production (Davis and Sinning, 1987). This finding is probably a more reliable indicator of potential motor problems in individuals with Down syndrome than the frequently cited link between hypotonia and motor problems (e.g. Morris, Vaughan and Vaccaro, 1982; Shepherd, 1980). It is feasible, therefore, that these children may be less accurate in controlling the force parameter in an ongoing and complex movement situation.

Summary

There is only limited information available on motor control of complex movements that allows comparisons to be made among normal, clumsy and intellectually disabled children on how they control and coordinate their movements. The majority of the motor control studies on exceptional populations have been conducted on children with Down syndrome performing relatively simple motor tasks. Other studies which have been reviewed in this section have shown an age-related improvement in children's movement speed for single-limbed tasks, and improvement in the timing parameters of a movement. Furthermore, studies on motor impaired children have indicated that children with Down syndrome may have deficiencies in controlling the timing and spatial parameters of a movement and, although they can set muscle length–tension ratios in a similar way to normal individuals, there is evidence to suggest that they would be unable to maintain accuracy of their movements. Thus, persons with Down syndrome appear to have underlying problems in motor control which would make it difficult for them to coordinate their movements. It should be noted though, that these findings have largely been derived from studies at ages older than those of the children who have participated in the study reported in this book.

Because of the lack of research in the control of complex movements in normally developing and motor impaired children, other than those with Down syndrome, the final sections in this chapter review pertinent literature on interlimb coordination in adults and children, and report research by the authors into how normally developing and motor impaired children control complex movements.

INTERLIMB BIMANUAL MOVEMENTS

Interlimb bimanual tasks involve coordinated movements in which two actions are performed simultaneously with separate hands. To reiterate the findings of the literature review from the previous section, current theories in motor control have hypothesized that movement is controlled at multiple levels within the central nervous system (e.g. Arbib, 1980, 1984; Glencross, 1980; Schmidt, 1988). An intermediate level of control is achieved by movement synergies (e.g. Easton, 1977; Lee, 1984), in which the movements are tuned by feedforward and feedback systems. The specifications for the movement appear to be derived from parameters which are best conceptualized as being part of a generalized motor programme. The parameters of a movement may be invariant, that is under higher order control, or variant if they are under more peripheral control. This would mean that any aspects of the movement which affect both limbs could be classified as invariant and should further our knowledge about constraints imposed by synergies in complex movements. Aspects of the movement which differ for each limb are considered variant and highlight the aspects of coordinated movement which are not constrained.

Tasks involving bimanual movements have been the subject of quite extensive research in the behavioural sciences (Corcos, 1984; Kelso *et al.*, 1981; Kelso, Putnam and Goodman, 1983; Kelso, Southard and Goodman, 1979a,b; Marteniuk and MacKenzie, 1980; Marteniuk, MacKenzie and Baba, 1984; Swinnen, 1990; Walter and Swinnen, 1992). Kelso and colleagues, and Marteniuk and MacKenzie, appear to have conducted the major early research in the area. They chose interlimb bimanual tasks to isolate aspects of interlimb coordination, and to examine the issue of how complex movements are coordinated.

Initially, interlimb paradigms, and more specifically bimanual tasks, were expected to show results similar to those predicted by a much cited law of human movement capacity, known as Fitts' (1954) law. Fitts derived this law by using a reciprocal tapping task, a pin transfer and a disc transfer task. Both the tasks involved serial movements over varied distances (amplitude), to varied size end points (width). Fitts found that with other variables held constant, as width decreased movement time increased, and similarly, as amplitude increased movement time increased.

In contrast, Kelso, Southard and Goodman (1979a, b), argued that these results demonstrated that interlimb movements are controlled by a coordinative structure (or synergy to use the terminology adopted in this book). The studies by Kelso, Putnam and Goodman (1983) confirmed the earlier findings that the two limbs act together as a functional synergy in terms of timing and kinematic factors. Nevertheless, they found that the hand performing the easier task slowed down to synchronize with the hand performing the harder task, although there was some evidence that both hands adjusted to adopt a 'common time scaling for two-handed movements' (Kelso, Putnam and Goodman, 1983, p. 354).

On the basis of neurophysiological data and as a result of these experiments Kelso and his colleagues hypothesized that, although the timing or phasing of a movement is apparently invariant, timing constraints may not originate at 'higher cortical levels but rather arise from the functionally autonomous structures, perhaps at the level of cerebellum or below' (Kelso, Putnam and Goodman, 1983, p. 370). In addition, they claimed there is evidence that muscular force may vary even though the timing constraints are apparently invariant.

Conversely, Marteniuk and MacKenzie (1980) and Marteniuk, MacKenzie and Baba (1984) did not find that the hands arrived simultaneously when moving to targets at different distances, in interlimb tasks. They did find though, that similar movements resulted in a similar time for each hand, although movements over different distances, and using styli of different weights resulted in the hands landing on the targets at different times. From their results they claimed that when two limbs are performing different tasks, both hands will leave the starting position virtually simultaneously, but they will not arrive at the targets at the same time.

According to Marteniuk and MacKenzie (1980) and Marteniuk, MacKenzie and Baba (1984) the discrepancy in arriving at the targets in asymmetrical tasks is due to hemispheric interference, resulting in inhibition and facilitation effects which will alter the movement time of each hand. Hemispheric interference should change the intensity (a term used by the authors in preference to time or force parameters), between the limbs. This interference would explain why Marteniuk and colleagues found, for example that when the right hand moved 30 cm and the left 10 cm, the hand moving 30 cm in this condition moved faster than when both hands moved 30 cm. A similar interference effect was found in the hand moving 10 cm with the other hand moving 30 cm, under this condition the hand moving 10 cm was slower than when both hands simultaneously moved 10 cm. According to Heuer (1985) the presence of an interference implies that the movements of both limbs are controlled by the same mechanism, so providing some support for the claims made by Marteniuk and colleagues.

Part of the discrepancy in results by these early researchers in interlimb bimanual tasks is that the research paradigms differ in distance requirement and in the required endpoint accuracy. The studies by Kelso and colleagues, for example, have far less stringent spatial accuracy requirements than the procedures of Marteniuk and colleagues. The interpretations of the research findings also differ because of the divergent theoretical assumptions held by the researchers. For instance, Kelso and colleagues favoured a mass-spring model and an oscillator system of motor control (Craske and Craske, 1986; Greene, 1982), whereas Marteniuk and colleagues were of the opinion that although their data support a model of motor control which acknowledges length–tension parameters, it also allowed for 'neural cross talk' between the hemispheres (Marteniuk, MacKenzie and Baba, 1984, p. 362).

The argument that there is neural cross-talk in dual task performance is strengthened by recent work by Swinnen *et al.* (1991a), who are of the opinion that symmetrical movements with both hands are no more difficult than a single limb movement. It is only when the movement of both upper limbs is asymmetrical that coordination and control become more difficult. This is because there appears to be a strong tendency to produce a synchronous movement pattern, particularly in the spatial and temporal requirements of a simultaneous bimanual task (Swinnen, 1990; Swinnen *et al.*, 1991b; Walter and Swinnen, 1992). In fact these authors have argued that seemingly very complex tasks may be relatively easier to perform than ones that appear simpler. This is because there is a tendency for the central nervous system to generate multi-limb movements, rather than trying to control two separate movements in parallel fashion.

The tendency towards synchrony in bimanual tasks has also been shown to occur in children aged 5 – 9 years (Fagard, 1987). It was found that in an interlimb bimanual cranking task children performed better when cranking at the same speed for each hand than a different speed with each hand. Such a finding would suggest that young children are more able to control symmetrical, than asymmetrical synchronous bimanual tasks. It was noted though, that the 9 year olds were better at controlling asymmetrical cranking movements than the younger children.

The reviewed research on interlimb bimanual coordination provides evidence of functional synergies which constrain movements of paired limbs, especially when they are moved simultaneously. This is because consistency in the timing of both hands has been reported by all researchers for symmetrical simultaneous movements. This tendency towards synchrony in bimanual movements could be interpreted as a neuromotor synergy (Lee, 1984). It also supports Lee's (1984) claim that bimanual interference between limbs is present in automatic and voluntary movements even when it is not essential for that particular movement task.

A STUDY OF THE INTERLIMB CONTROL OF MOTOR IMPAIRED CHILDREN

The study reported in this chapter, on interlimb coordination in normally developing and motor impaired children, represents an attempt to establish the manner in which children control a relatively complex coordination task. As such it redresses in part the lack of research into the motor control processes in normally developing and motor impaired children, in early and middle childhood. The thrust of the study was also to ascertain if there were any underlying differences in motor control, which might help to explain the differences which have been found in the motor performance and fundamental movement patterns of normally developing, clumsy and intellectually disabled children and children with Down syndrome. In fact motor control studies should provide the theoretical perspective to explain why some of the frequently observed differences actually occur.

Having validated the procedures in three previous studies (O'Brien, 1988) this study sought to determine whether motor impaired children (specifically, children who are clumsy or intellectually disabled and children who have Down syndrome) control their upper limbs in a similar fashion to that of normally developing children. It is apparent from the literature that has already been reported that bimanual movements are controlled as a movement synergy, within which timing and muscle length–tension ratios are similar for symmetrical movements and are modified by bilateral inhibition in asymmetrical movements. Moreover, earlier studies by O'Brien (1988) indicated that younger children (6 years of age) are not able to formulate or control their interlimb movements as competently as children in middle childhood (10 year olds) and adults.

RESULTS OF THE STUDY OF TIMING AND ACCURACY FACTORS IN INTERLIMB CONTROL OF MOTOR IMPAIRED CHILDREN

The specific measures in this study were response time, movement time, total movement time and spatial accuracy. Methods, Procedures and Results are reported in detail in Appendix C.

Response time

The response time data (response time represented the time taken to initiate a movement response after an auditory signal), would seem to indicate that clumsy, intellectually disabled and children with Down syndrome have a slower response processing time than normally developing children. Such a finding suggests that all these motor impaired children take longer to organize a movement response than normally developing peers. Furthermore, the results from the study, in part, refute what appears to be merely a delay in development in the intellectually disabled children who were found to be significantly slower in response speed than children who are normally developing or clumsy and children with Down syndrome. The response time results also appear to contradict findings reported in the literature that have suggested that children with Down syndrome have a slower reaction time than intellectually disabled peers (Henderson, 1985). Perhaps the apparent discrepancy in the results between the present and previous studies is due to the fact that more complex movement tasks were used, which measured the time it took to organize a movement response instead of a reaction time to a sensory stimulus (Hoover and Wade, 1985).

The response time results of the intellectually disabled children may help to explain why these children have frequently been described as slow in their movements (e.g. Connolly and Michael, 1986; Hoover and Wade, 1985). It would appear that they take longer than the other groups of motor impaired children to organize their movement responses especially for movements further away form their body. Such movements are probably a more complex task than movements closer to the body (Christina and Rose, 1985), and so emphasize the deficit and consequential slowness that intellectually disabled children have in organizing their movements.

A further finding from the response-time data was that the difference between the younger and older groups of clumsy children was greater than for the other motor impaired groups. This suggests that response organization in younger clumsy children is more of a deficit in this age range than it is in normally developing, intellectually disabled and Down syndrome children. Moreover, this finding may explain some of the previously noted marked age discrepancies in movement patterns and motor performance (Chapters 3–5) between the younger and older clumsy children. The assumption is that the accelerated motor development, in comparison with other motor impaired children may, in part, be related to an increased ability to organize movement responses as they grow older. Of interest also from the response time data, was the fact that children with Down syndrome did not exhibit as marked a deficit in organizing a movement response as their intellectually disabled peers.

Movement time

The movement-time data (i.e. speed of the actual movement, once the movement is initiated) showed that 6 year olds moved their upper limbs at a slower speed than 10 year olds. In regard to speed of movement, the results from this study suggest that normal and clumsy children had a similar movement time, whereas children with Down syndrome had a significantly slower movement time than either normal, clumsy or intellectually disabled children. Such a finding helps explain the previously observed slowness in movement in these children (e.g. Connolly and Michael, 1986). The reason for their slowness, unlike their intellectually disabled peers, appears to be not so much in their ability to organize a movement response, but in their slowness at actually executing the movement. The results also showed that the speed of movement of children with Down syndrome had a proportionally greater age-related change than the other groups, whereas age-related rate of change in speed stays relatively constant for intellectually disabled, clumsy and normally developing children.

Total movement time

For total movement time (i.e. response time plus movement time), the data indicated that younger children were once again significantly slower than the older children. In addition all the children were slower when moving 10 cm than when moving 30 cm. Unlike the movement-time data there was a significant time discrepancy when both hands moved 10 and 30 cm when compared with the hands moving unequal distances (10(Left):30(Right) or 30(Left):10(Right)). In these results normally developing children were significantly faster than the motor impaired children, and clumsy children were significantly faster than children with intellectual disability or Down syndrome, who did not differ significantly from each other. This means that normally developing children would be expected to move faster to achieve specified movement goals than the other children, and it may again help to explain the reports that children with intellectual disability and Down syndrome move slowly (e.g. Connolly and Michael, 1986).

Spatial accuracy

In the spatial accuracy measure (how close the children were to hitting the centre of the target plate with each hand), 6 year olds were less accurate than 10 year olds and all the children were more accurate when they moved 10 cm rather than 30 cm. There was evidence of asymmetry in spatial accuracy because when the hands moved an equal distance the accuracy was better than when the hands moved different distances. Moving different distances was more difficult for all the children, irrespective of category. The spatial accuracy results indicated that accuracy and hence muscle length–tension ratios were easier to achieve in the right hand than the left hand, and that there was asymmetry in this aspect of movement control.

The reported study of motor control has identified factors in response time, movement time and total movement time, which may help to explain some of the observed differences in movement behaviour among normally developing children, those who are clumsy, intellectually disabled and with Down syndrome.

SUMMARY OF THE STUDY

In summary this study has indicated the following.

1. There is some evidence from the timing and spatial accuracy data of bilateral inhibition and, hence, a tendency to produce a synchronous movement pattern when children move two hands simultaneously to targets of unequal distance, in a specified movement task.
2. The asymmetry noted in the spatial accuracy data would suggest that it is easier for all the children to set precise muscle length–tension ratios for the right hand rather than the left hand, in the age groups and categories of children who participated in this experiment.
3. Clumsy children had a proportionally greater change between 6 and 10 years of age in response organization in comparison with children who are normally developing, intellectually disabled and children who have Down syndrome. It is suggested that this may reflect the higher cognitive ability of the clumsy children when compared to their intellectually disabled peers or children with Down syndrome.
4. Intellectually disabled children had greater problems in organizing both hands to move different distances than the children who are normally developing, clumsy and with Down syndrome. This may constitute an interlimb bilateral organization deficit.
5. If response time is regarded as the time taken to organize a movement response then intellectually disabled children would be expected to be slower than the other groups of children. Normally developing children were the fastest and children who were clumsy and children with Down syndrome are similar in their response speed.
6. Children with Down syndrome had a slower movement speed than normal, clumsy and intellectually disabled children. This slowness may be partly due to their muscular hypotonia, and also an inability voluntarily to set muscular stiffness when compared with the other groups of children.
7. Normally developing children were significantly faster in total movement time than children who are clumsy, intellectually disabled or with Down syndrome, also the clumsy children were faster than the intellectually disabled

group. Again this finding may explain why children with intellectual disability or Down syndrome appear to move so slowly.

8. There is evidence that younger normally developing children were faster at formulating response parameters, moved at a greater speed and achieved movement tasks quicker and more accurately than children who are clumsy and intellectually disabled and children with Down syndrome, of the same age.

CONCLUSION

It is apparent that the interlimb bimanual study reported here has revealed that motor impaired children, in general, have underlying control problems which will affect their movement skills. Specifically, the findings of slower response times in intellectually disabled children, and slower movement times in children with Down syndrome explains, in part, the observable slowness of movement in these two groups of children. Additionally, the lower motor performance scores of younger clumsy children, in comparison with the older group of clumsy children may partly be explained by their comparatively less efficient motor control processes. The implications for practice of these results, together with the results from the sections on motor performance and fundamental movement patterns, will be discussed in the next chapter.

REFERENCES

Abernathy, B. and Sparrow, W.A. (1992) The rise and fall of dominant paradigms in motor behaviour research, in *Approaches to the Study of Motor Control and Learning*, (ed. J.J. Summers), Elsevier Science, Amsterdam, pp. 3–43.

Arbib, M.A. (1980) Interacting schemas for motor control, in *Tutorials in Motor Behavior* (eds G.E. Stelmach and J.E. Requin), North-Holland, Amsterdam, pp. 71–82.

Arbib, M.A. (1984) From synergies and embryos to motor schemas, in *Human Motor Actions: Bernstein Reassessed* (ed. H.T.A. Whiting), North Holland, Elsevier Science, Amsterdam, pp. 545–62.

Bernstein, N. (1967) *The Coordination and Regulation of Movements*, Pergamon, London.

Brown, J.M.M. and Parker, A.W. (1992) Comparison of gait in five to seven year-old children. *Journal of Human Movement Studies*, **22**, 101–15.

Burton, A.W. (1986) The effect of age on relative timing variability and transfer. *Journal of Motor Behavior*, **18**, 323–42.

Burton, A.W. (1987) The effect of number of movement components on response time in children. *Journal of Motor Behavior*, **13**, 231–47.

Charlton, J.L. (1992) Motor control considerations for assessment and rehabilitation of movement disorders, in *Approaches to the Study of Motor Control and Learning*, (ed. J.J. Summers), North Holland, Elsevier Science, Amsterdam, pp. 3–43.

Christina, R.W. and Rose, D.J. (1985) Premotor and motor reaction time as a function of response complexity. *Research Quarterly for Exercise and Sport*, **56**, 306–15.

Clark, J.E. (1982) The role of response mechanisms in motor skill development, in *The Development of Movement Control and Co-ordination*, (eds J.A.S. Kelso and J.E. Clark), John Wiley, Chichester, pp. 151–73.

Clark, J.E. and Whitall, J. (1989) Changing patterns of locomotion: from walking to skipping, in *Development of Posture and Gait Across the Life Span*, (eds M.H. Woollacott and A. Shumway-Cook), University of Southern California, Columbia, pp. 128–51.

Colley, A.M. and Beech, J.R. (1988) Grounds for reconciliation: some preliminary thoughts on cognition and action, in *Cognition and Action in Skilled Behavior* (eds A.M. Colley and J.R. Beech), Elsevier Science, Amsterdam, pp. 397–403.

Connolly, K. (1980) The development of competence in motor skills, in *Scientific Foundations of Developmental Psychiatry* (ed. M. Rutter), William Heinemann, London, pp. 138–53.

Connolly, K.J. (1986) A perspective on motor development, in *Motor Development in Children: Aspects of Coordination and Control* (eds M.G. Wade and H.T.A. Whiting), Martinus Nijhoff, Dordrecht, pp. 3–21.

Connolly, B.H. and Michael, B.T. (1986) Performance of retarded children with and without Down's Syndrome, on the Bruininks–Oseretsky Test of Motor Proficiency. *Physical Therapy*, **66**, 344–8.

Corcos, D.M. (1984) Two-handed movement control. *Research Quarterly for Exercise and Sport*, **55**, 117–22.

Craske, B. and Craske, J.D. (1986) Oscillator mechanisms in the human motor system: investigating their properties using the after contraction effect. *Journal of Motor Behavior*, **18**, 117–45.

Davis, W.E. and Kelso, J.A.S. (1982) Analysis of 'invariant characteristics' in the motor control of Down's Syndrome and normal subjects. *Journal of Motor Behavior*, **14**, 194–212.

Davis, W.E. and Sinning, W.E. (1987) Muscle stiffness in Down Syndrome and other mentally handicapped subjects: a research role. *Journal of Motor Behavior*, **19**, 130–44.

Deitz, V. (1992) Human neuronal control of automatic functional movements: interaction between central programs and afferent input. *Physiological Reviews*, **72**, 33–69.

Easton, T.A. (1977) Coordinative structures: the basis for a motor program, in *Psychology of Motor Behavior and Sport* (eds D.M. Landers and R.W. Christina), Human Kinetics, Champaign, IL, pp. 3–90.

Fagard, J. (1987) Bimanual stereotypes: bimanual coordination in children as a function of age. *Journal of Motor Behavior*, **19**, 355–66.

Ferrandez, A.M. and Pailhouse, J. (1986) A note on modulations and structuring of locomotion in children and adults. *Journal of Motor Behavior*, **18**, 475–85.

Fitts, P.M. (1954) The information capacity of the human motor system in controlling the amplitude of movement. *Journal of Experimental Psychology*, **47**, 381–91.

Frith, U. and Frith, C.D. (1974) Specific motor disabilities in Down's Syndrome. *Journal of Child Psychology and Psychiatry*, **15**, 293–301.

Gallagher, J.D. and Thomas, J.R. (1986) Developmental effects of grouping and recoding on learning a movement series. *Research Quarterly for Exercise and Sport*, **57**, 117–27.

Glencross, D.J. (1980) Levels and strategies of response organization, in *Tutorials in Motor Behavior* (eds G.E. Stelmach and J. Requin), North Holland, Amsterdam, pp. 551–6.

Greene, P.H. (1982) Why is it easy to control your arms? *Journal of Motor Behavior*, **14**, 260–86.

Guiard, Y. (1987) Asymmetric division of labor in human bimanual action: the kinematic chain as a model. *Journal of Motor Behavior*, **19**, 486–517.

Henderson, S.E. (1985) Motor skill development, in *Current Approaches to Down's Syndrome* (eds D. Lane and B. Stratford), Holt, Rinehart and Winston, London, pp. 187–213.

Heuer, H. (1985) Intermanual interaction during simultaneous execution and programming of finger movements. *Journal of Motor Behavior*, **17**, 325–34.

Hinton, G. (1984) Parallel computations for controlling an arm. *Journal of Motor Behavior*, **16**, 171–94.

Hogg, J. and Moss, S.N. (1983) Prehensile development in Down's Syndrome and non-handicapped preschool children. *British Journal of Developmental Psychology*, **1**, 189–204.

Hoover, J.H. and Wade, M.G. (1985) Motor learning theory. *Adapted Physical Activity Quarterly*, **2**, 228–52.

Ivry, R.B. (1986) Force and timing components of the motor program. *Journal of Motor Behavior*, **18**, 449–74.

Keele, S.W. (1981) Behavioral analysis of movement, in *Handbook of Physiology, Section 1: The Nervous System, Vol II, Motor Control, Part 2* (ed. V.B. Brooks), American Physiological Society, Baltimore, pp. 1391–414.

Keele, S.W., Ivry, R.I. and Pokorny, R.A. (1987) Force control and its relation to timing. *Journal of Motor Behavior*, **19**, 96–114.

Kelso, J.A.S., Holt, K.G., Rubin, P. and Kugler, P.N. (1981) Patterns of human interlimb coordination emerge from the properties of non-linear, limit cycle oscillatory processes: theory and data. *Journal of Motor Behavior*, **31**, 226–61.

Kelso, J.A.S., Putnam, C.A. and Goodman, D. (1983) On the space time structure of human interlimb co-ordination. *Quarterly Journal of Experimental Psychology*, **35A**, 347–75.

Kelso, J.A.S., Southard, D.L. and Goodman, D. (1979a) On the coordination of two-handed movements. *Journal of Experimental Psychology: Human Perception and Performance*, **5**, 229–38.

Kelso, J.A.S., Southard, D.L. and Goodman, D. (1979b) On the nature of human interlimb coordination. *Science*, **203**, 1029–31.

Keogh, J. and Sugden, D. (1985) *Movement Skill Development*, Macmillan, New York.

Lee, W.A. (1984) Neuromotor synergies as a basis for coordinated intentional action. *Journal of Motor Behavior*, **16**, 135–70.

Marteniuk, R.G. and MacKenzie, C.L. (1980) A preliminary theory of two-handed control, in *Tutorials in Motor Behavior* (eds G.E. Stelmach and J. Requin), North Holland, Amsterdam, pp. 185–97.

Marteniuk, R.G., MacKenzie, C.L. and Baba, D.M. (1984) Bimanual movement control: information processing and interaction effects. *Quarterly Journal of Experimental Psychology*, **36A**, 335–65.

Morris, A.F., Vaughan, S.E. and Vaccaro, P. (1982) Measurements of neuromuscular tone and strength in Down's Syndrome children. *Journal of Mental Deficiency Research*, **26**, 41–6.

Mounoud, P. (1986) Action and cognition: cognitive and motor skills in a developmental perspective, in *Motor Development in Children: Aspects of Coordination and Control* (eds M.G. Wade and H.T.A. Whiting), Martinus Nijhoff, Dordrecht, pp. 373–90.

Newell, K.M. (1980) The speed–accuracy paradox in movement control: errors of time and space, in *Tutorials in Motor Behavior* (eds G.E. Stelmach and J. Requin), North Holland, Amsterdam, pp. 501–10.

Newell, K.M., Morris, L.R. and Scully, D.M. (1985) Augmented information and the acquisition of skill in physical activity. *Exercise and Sport Sciences Reviews*, **13**, 235–61.

O'Brien, C.C. (1988) Motor development in clumsy, intellectually disabled and Down's syndrome children: a comparative study. Unpublished PhD thesis, University of Queensland.

Patla, A.E. (1985) Some characteristics of E.M.G. patterns during locomotion: implications for the locomotor control process. *Journal of Motor Behavior*, **17**, 443–61.

Reed, E.S. (1982) An outline of a theory of action systems. *Journal of Motor Behavior*, **14**, 98–134.

Roberton, M.A. and Halverson, L.E. (1988) The development of locomotor co-ordination: longitudinal change and invariance. *Journal of Motor Behavior*, **20**, 197–241.

Schellekens, J.M.H., Kalverboer, A.F. and Scholten, C.A. (1984) The microstructure of tapping movements in children. *Journal of Motor Behavior*, **16**, 20–39.

Schmidt, R.A. (1980) On the theoretical status of time in motor program representations in *Tutorials in Motor Behavior* (eds G.E. Stelmach and J. Requin), North-Holland, Amsterdam, pp. 146–65.

Schmidt, R.A. (1988) *Motor Control and Learning*, Human Kinetics, Champaign, Il.

Seyfort, B. and Spreen, O. (1979) Two-plated tapping performance by Down's Syndrome and non-Down's Syndrome retardates. *Journal of Child Psychology and Psychiatry*, **20**, 351–55.

Shapiro, D.C., Zernicke, R.F., Gregor, R.J. and Diestel, J.D. (1981) Evidence for a generalized motor program using gait pattern analysis. *Journal of Motor Behavior*, **13**, 33–47.

Shepherd, R.B. (1980) Problem analysis with Down's Syndrome infants. *Cumberland College Reports*, **20**, 1–14.

Shik, M.L. and Orlovsky, G.N. (1976) Neurophysiology of locomotor automatism. *Physiological Reviews*, **56**, 465–501.

Smyth, M.M. (1986) Relating cognition and action: reaction to Mounoud, in *Motor Development in Children: Aspects of Coordination and Control* (eds M.G. Wade and H.T.A. Whiting), Martinus Nijhoff, Dordrecht, pp. 391–403.

Smyth, T.R. (1991) Abnormal clumsiness in children: a defect of motor programming? *Child Care, Health and Development*, **17**, 283–94.

Smyth, T.R. (1992) Impaired motor skill (clumsiness) in otherwise normal children: a review. *Child Care, Health and Development*, **18**, 283–300.

Sparrow, W.A. (1983) The efficiency of skilled performance. *Journal of Motor Behavior*, **3**, 237–61.

Stelmach, E. and Diggles, V.A. (1982) Control theories in motor behavior. *Acta Psychologica*, **50**, 83–105.

Summers, J.J. (1975) The role of timing in motor program representation. *Journal of Motor Behavior*, **7**, 229–42.

Swinnen, S.P. (1990) *Journal of Experimental Psychology: Learning, Memory and Cognition*, **16**, 692–705.

Swinnen, S.P. and Walter, C.B. (1991) Toward a movement dynamics perspective on dual-task performance. *Human Factors*, **33**, 367–87.

Swinnen, S.P., Beirinckx, M.B., Meugens, P.F. and Walter, C.B. (1991a) Dissociating the structural and metrical specifications of bimanual movement. *Journal of Motor Behavior*, **23**, 263–79.

Swinnen, S.P., Young, D.E., Walter, C.B. and Serrien, D.J. (1991b) Control of asymmetrical bimanual movements. *Experimental Brain Research*, **85**, 163–73.

Turvey, M.T. and Kugler, P.N. (1984) An ecological approach to perception and action, in *Tutorials in Motor Behavior* (eds G.E. Stelmach and J.E. Requin), North-Holland, Amsterdam, pp. 373–412.

Turvey, M.T., Shaw, R.E. and Mace, W. (1978) Issues in the theory of action, degrees of freedom, coordinative structures and coalitions. *Attention and Performance*, **7**, 557–95.

Viviani, P. and Terzuolo, C. (1980) Space–time invariance in learned motor skills, in *Tutorials in Motor Behavior* (eds G.E. Stelmach and J.E. Requin), North-Holland, Amsterdam, pp. 523–33.

Walter, C.B. and Swinnen, S.P. (1992) Active tuning of interlimb attraction to facilitate bimanual decoupling. *Journal of Motor Behavior*, **24**, 95–104.

Whiting, H.T.A., Vogt, S. and Vereijken, B. (1992) Human skills and motor control–motor learning relation, in *Approaches to the Study of Motor Control and Learning* (ed. J.J. Summers), Elsevier, Science, Amsterdam, pp. 81–111.

Winter, D.A. (1983) Biomechanical motor patterns in normal walking. *Journal of Motor Behavior*, **15**, 302–30.

7

Summary, implications and conclusions from the present studies: recommendations for physical activity programmes

Motor development was examined in this book in terms of a movement hierarchy and from a neurobehavioural perspective which identified some of the sensory-neurological, integrative-perceptual, motor control processes considered to influence movement behaviour of normally developing children. Using this neurobehavioural perspective a major contribution of this book has been in the development and testing of multiple measures of movement behaviour, to be used both with normal and motor impaired children. These measures have provided important information for the investigation of motor impairment and for the development of guidelines for adapted motor programmes.

SUMMARY OF THE APPROACH TO MOVEMENT BEHAVIOUR ADOPTED IN THE BOOK

The observable changes in movement behaviour, described in the movement hierarchy, were conceptualized as progressing from very little control over movement, to some control, to very precise control. Early movement patterns were viewed as being controlled largely by basic processes and complex skills as being performed mainly by using advanced processes. The neurobehavioural perspective identified sensory systems and muscle tone as important sensory-neurological processes; sensory integration and postural stability as examples of integrative-perceptual processes. Examples of motor learning-control processes were information processing and the control of spatial, timing and force parameters of movement. A review of previous research on how these processes affect motor impaired children showed that a combination of deficiencies in these processes was likely to be the cause of the observed differences in the motor behaviour of children who are clumsy or intellectually disabled and children with Down syndrome.

The literature which has been reported in previous chapters suggests that those clumsy children found to have movement problems as babies, maintained these problems throughout early childhood. Clumsy children were also reported to exhibit many sensory-neurological and integrative-perceptual processes which would be likely to interfere with control of movement. For instance, many of these children, particularly those under 10 years of age, were reported to have movement problems, in the form of sensory processing dysfunction, neurological 'soft signs' such as jerky, irregular, poorly timed movements, delayed laterality and generalized lack of strength. Cognitive problems were inferred from reported difficulties, in some of these children, in processing visual and kinaesthetic information, formulating distance and spatial relationships, and in planning and executing movements.

Intellectually disabled children appear to differ from normally developing children, particularly in sensory-neurological processes, as they have been shown to have delayed postural reflexes, muscle tone abnormalities, and poor body awareness. Furthermore, research evidence has demonstrated delays in integrative-perceptual processes since their sensory integration ability is similar to children of the same mental rather than chronological age. In terms of advanced processes, intellectually disabled children have deficits in information processing and more specifically, a slower reaction time, which is a measure of the speed with which they can initiate a motor response.

Children with Down syndrome have been shown to have deficiencies in nearly all areas associated with sensory-neurological processes. They maintain primitive reflexes for a longer period than normally developing children, show generalized hypotonia (low muscle tone), and exhibit delayed postural reflex development. It also has been found that they have deficiencies in integrative-perceptual processes. For example, they do not process vestibular, visual and auditory sensory information in the same way as other groups of children. The motor learning-control processing problems of children with Down syndrome include deficits in short-term memory and storage, and retrieval of sensory information, particularly visual and kinaesthetic information. In addition, they appear to have problems in formulating motor programmes and in controlling the timing and force of their movements.

The literature review, therefore, indicated that motor impaired children who are clumsy, intellectually disabled or who have Down syndrome are likely to have specific problems, in basic, intermediate and advanced movement control processes, integrative and cognitive processes that assist them in controlling their movements, and that these problems differ among the groups and categories of the motor impaired children who participated in the studies that have been reported in this book.

However, it was not possible from the literature to gain a comprehensive picture of the motor problems for each of the categories of children that were studied. This was because most of the previous research has tended to assess children's development by measuring only one dimension of the particular behaviour, and as already stated, the impression of delay or difference is dependent on the method of assessment (Chapter 2). For example, norm-referenced performance scores for a particular child can only be interpreted in terms of whether their score is above or below the 'normal' score for their age or grade. In order to overcome the problems associated with use of a single measure of assessment, three different measures were chosen to examine movement behaviour, these were motor performance, fundamental movement patterns and interlimb motor control. The advantages and disadvantages of each of these measures were discussed in Chapter 2.

Table 7.1 Summary of significant differences in multiple-measures of movement behaviour in groups of motor impaired children

Motor performance

- All motor impaired children obtained a lower score than their BOT-S age norms.
- All motor impaired groups had lower scores in early than in middle childhood.
- (C), in comparison with other motor impaired children, showed a different rate of progress.

Early childhood

- (C) scored higher in catching than (ID) and (DS).
- (C) faster than (DS) in agility run.
- (C) same as (ID) in agility run, bilateral coordination, catching and throwing for accuracy.
- (C), (ID) and (DS) had similar scores in static balance, bilateral coordination, and standing broad jump.
- (C) lower score than (ID) and (DS) in dynamic balance.

Middle childhood

- (C) obtained higher scores in static and dynamic balance than (ID) and (DS).
- (C) faster than (ID) and (DS) in agility run.
- (C), (ID), and (DS) obtained similar scores in bilateral coordination, catching and throwing for accuracy.

Movement patterns

- Total fundamental pattern scores were highest for (N), then (C), then (ID) and (DS) in descending order.
- The pattern of change differed, according to the age and category of the children.

Early childhood

- (N) had more mature walking and running profiles than (C).

Middle childhood

- (N) exhibited higher levels of maturity in their profiles than (C).

- (C) had more mature walking, running, jumping, throwing and catching profiles than (ID) and (DS).
- (C), (ID) and (DS), as a group are almost one level more mature in their locomotor than their manipulative skills.

- (C) and (ID) have similar walking and running profiles.
- (C) had more mature jumping, throwing and catching profiles than (ID) and (DS).
- (ID) and (DS) had similar jumping, throwing and catching profiles.

Motor control

- All categories of children were faster in middle than in early childhood, in measures of response time, movement time and total movement time.
- The pattern of results differed according to the category of the children.
- There was a similar pattern for each category at each age level (unlike the other measures). Therefore, the results are reported for both age groups together.

- All children obtained similar results in measures of spatial accuracy.
- (N) were faster than (C), then (ID) and (DS) respectively, in total movement time.
- (N) were faster in response time measures than (C), (ID) and (DS).
- (C) and (DS) were faster in response time measures than (ID).
- (N), (C) and (ID) had faster movement time than (DS).

Abbreviations: (N) = normally developing children; (C) = clumsy children; (ID) = intellectually disabled children; (DS) = Down syndrome children.

SUMMARY OF THE RESULTS OF THE MOVEMENT BEHAVIOUR STUDIES IN CHILDREN WHO ARE NORMALLY DEVELOPING, CLUMSY, INTELLECTUALLY DISABLED AND WITH DOWN SYNDROME

The results from the studies using the three measures separately to examine motor performance, fundamental movement patterns and interlimb coordination, are reported in this section.

Motor performance

In terms of motor performance all the groups of motor impaired children progressed in a similar way, but obtained test scores lower than those reported for normally developing children. Younger motor impaired children were significantly lower in performance than older peers on subtests measuring running speed and agility, static balance, jump and clap, standing broad jump, catching and throwing for accuracy. In the younger age group clumsy children were superior in catching to their intellectually disabled and Down syndrome peers, and ran

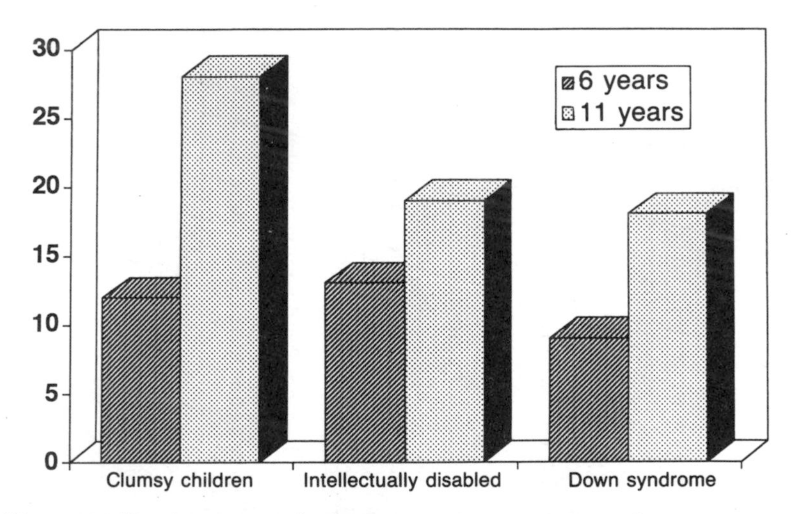

Figure 7.1 Total scores on the Bruininks–Oseretsky Test of Motor Proficiency (Short Form).

faster than children with Down syndrome. In contrast, younger children who are clumsy, intellectually disabled or have Down syndrome, obtained similar scores on items measuring static balance, bilateral coordination and standing broad jump. Of particular interest was the fact that the clumsy children scored lower than the other motor impaired groups in the dynamic balance task.

Older clumsy children scored significantly higher in the running speed and agility than their intellectually disabled peers, and intellectually disabled children were faster than children with Down syndrome. In bilateral coordination, as assessed by catching and throwing, the scores obtained by the different categories of children were similar (Figure 7.1 and Table 7.1 give a summary of results).

FUNDAMENTAL MOVEMENT PATTERNS

All the groups of motor impaired children exhibited lower levels in their fundamental movement profiles than normal peers. Younger normally developing children had more mature walking and running profiles than clumsy age peers. The younger clumsy children demonstrated walking, running, jumping, catching and throwing patterns which were more mature than the younger children who were intellectually disabled or with Down syndrome.

By middle childhood the group of normally developing children had reached relatively mature levels of walking, running, jumping, catching and throwing, but not necessarily the most mature levels of these patterns. They were more mature, however, in all their fundamental movement profiles than children who were clumsy, intellectually disabled or had Down syndrome. Clumsy and intellectually disabled children had similar walking and running profiles, but the clumsy children had more mature jumping, catching and throwing patterns than intellectually disabled and the children with Down syndrome. The intellectually disabled children and children with Down syndrome had similar developmental levels in their jumping, catching and throwing.

Across ages there appeared to be a hierarchy of progression in the fundamental movement patterns. The results confirmed the value of the Fundamental Movement Pattern check-lists as a measure of developmental status both in normal and motor impaired children. Furthermore, the present project provided preliminary, cross-sectional, evidence that different categories of motor impaired children progressed through the hierarchy at different rates (Figure 7.2 and Table 7.1 give summaries of results).

Motor control

With regard to the motor control processes, as measured by response time, movement time, total movement time and spatial accuracy for a bimanual task, the results indicated that all the motor impaired children were slower and less accurate when the younger group was compared with the older group. It was found, however, that all the categories and age groups obtained similar scores on the spatial accuracy task. The results also indicated that normally developing children were faster in their response time and total movement time than the other motor impaired children. There were, however, differences on the separate measures of response time, movement time and total movement time in the different categories of motor impaired children. For example, in response time intellectually disabled children were significantly slower than children who

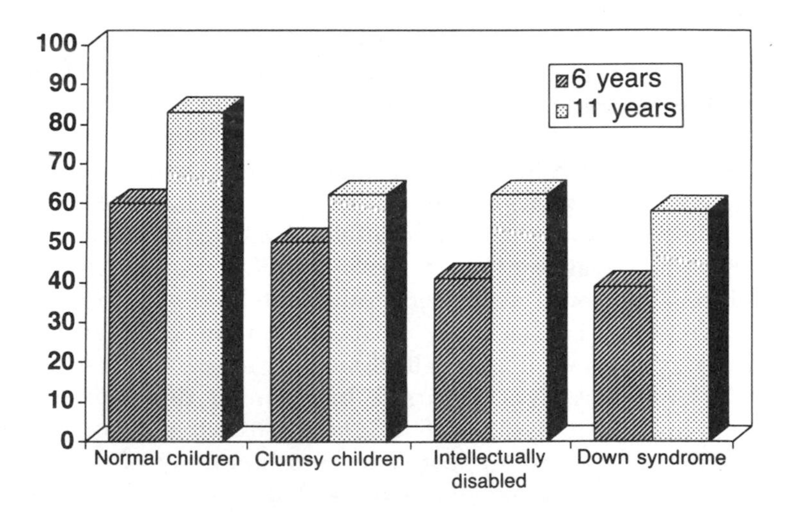

Figure 7.2 Total scores for fundamental movement patterns.

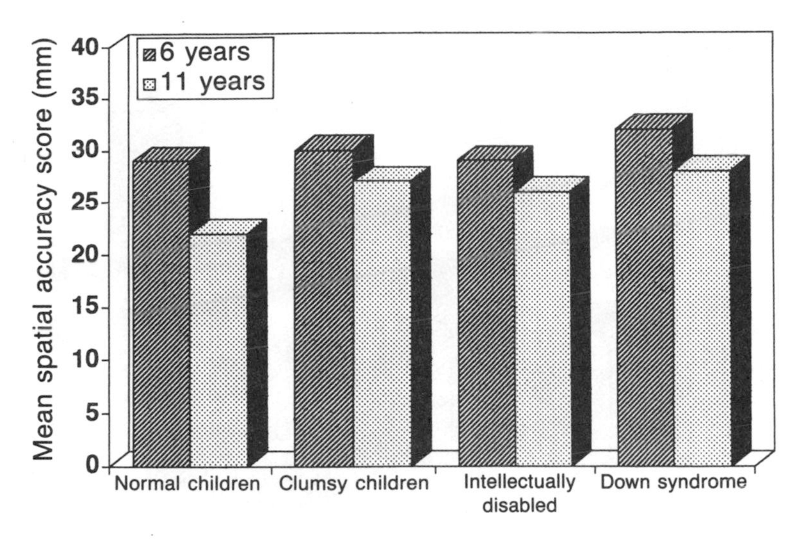

Figure 7.3 Mean spatial accuracy scores.

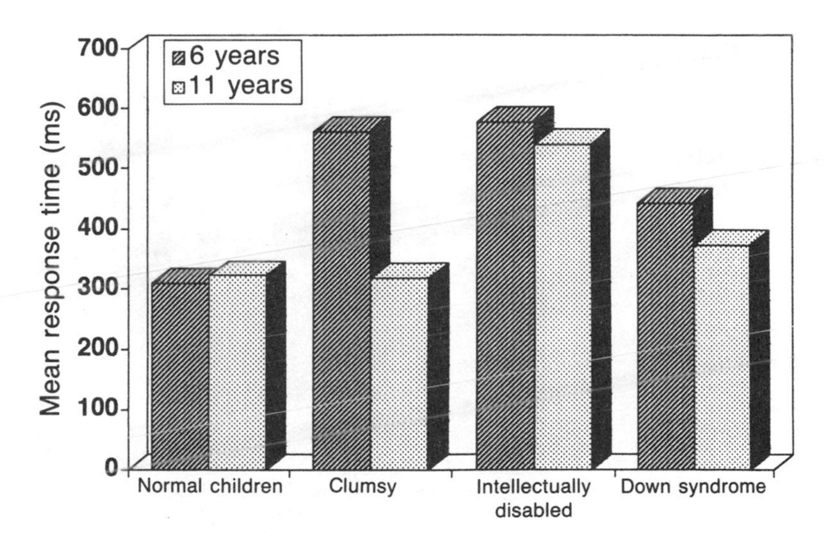

Figure 7.4 Mean response time.

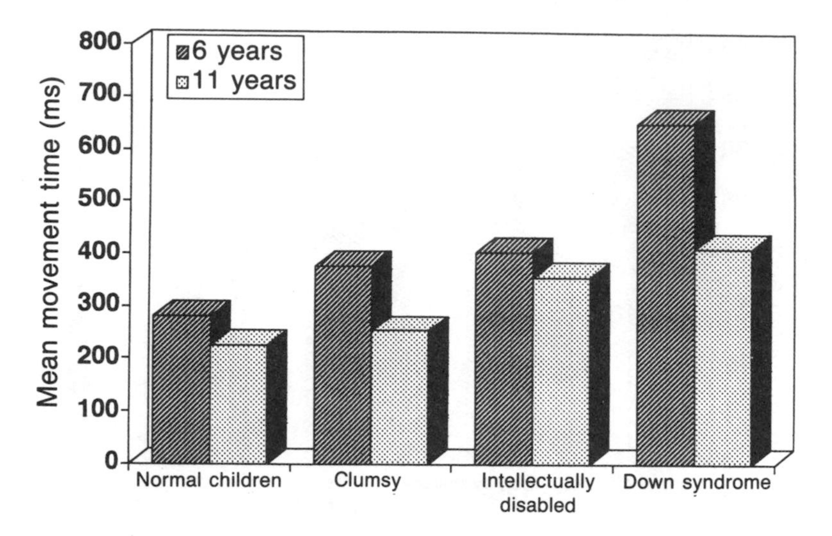

Figure 7.5 Mean movement time.

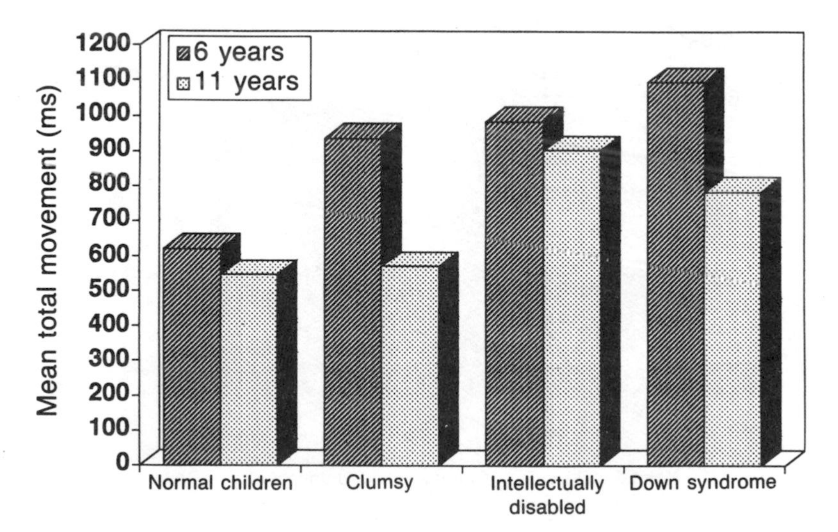

Figure 7.6 Mean total movement time.

are clumsy and children with Down syndrome had significantly slower movement times than the other motor impaired children (Figures 7.3–7.6 and Table 7.1 give summaries of the results).

IMPLICATIONS OF THE RESULTS FROM THE MEASURES OF MOVEMENT BEHAVIOUR IN CHILDREN WHO ARE DEVELOPING NORMALLY, CLUMSY, INTELLECTUALLY DISABLED OR WHO HAVE DOWN SYNDROME

The results from the three aspects of movement behaviour show an interesting pattern of similarities and differences among children who are normally developing, clumsy or intellectually disabled and those children with Down syndrome. The findings suggest that the children in the different categories appear to progress through predictable sequences of movement behaviours, which become more complex with increased age. The results, however, reveal that the way in which these groups of children progress is related to their impairment.

As suspected, the impression of delay or difference formed by the examiner is influenced by the measures of motor behaviour being used. For instance, from the motor performance measures, those who are intellectually disabled and children with Down syndrome would be classified as developmentally delayed, because they obtained consistently lower motor performance scores, both in early and middle childhood, than normally developing children. Clumsy children, in contrast, appeared to differ in their measures of motor performance more than the two other motor impaired groups. For example, younger clumsy children scored significantly lower on the dynamic balance item and no better than the younger children with intellectual disability or Down syndrome, on any of the other measures apart from catching. In contrast the older clumsy children were superior to the other two motor impaired groups in all items which assessed motor performance.

The fundamental movement profiles revealed both similarities and differences in the movement behaviour of motor impaired children. For instance, there are indications of similarities, in that all the motor impaired children have lower levels in their fundamental movement patterns than normally developing children. Children with Down syndrome, however, are more delayed than intellectually disabled children, who are more delayed than clumsy children. Differences are apparent in the clumsy children whose fundamental movement pattern levels appear to undergo an increased rate of improvement between early and middle childhood, than their motor impaired peers. The magnitude of delay, however, is constant in the intellectually disabled children. There is also evidence of differences in development, particularly in elements of the fundamental movement patterns in children with Down syndrome. These children appear to have a discrepancy in levels of maturity between the action of their upper and lower limbs. This discrepancy is evident in the walking, running and jumping patterns of children with Down syndrome.

When motor control processes are examined, yet another pattern of results emerges. Collectively, in early childhood the motor impaired groups are slower in terms of response time, movement time and total movement time, and they are less accurate in the control of the spatial parameters of a task. Once again, however, there are different patterns of results across the groups of motor impaired children.

The differences which were found were dependent on the measure used and the category of the children. For example, in terms of response time the intellectually disabled children were significantly slower than younger and older children who are clumsy or have Down syndrome. Additionally, in clumsy children the ratio of increase in response time between the younger and older groups was significantly greater, in comparison with their other motor impaired peers.

For children with Down syndrome a different pattern emerged in the results of the movement time measure. Although the response time measures appear to confirm that these children were able to respond to sensory input and organized a movement faster than their intellectually disabled peers, and as fast as clumsy peers, the movement time results indicated that they were significantly slower than the other motor impaired children in their movement time to complete a task. Additionally, the movement time results indicated that clumsy and normal children were found to move as fast as one another and faster than the intellectually disabled children. If response time and movement time were the only measures taken to assess motor impaired children, then the intellectually disabled children and those with Down syndrome would probably be classified as differing from normal motor development.

The total movement time results present another picture. The results of this measure seem to suggest that all motor impaired children are developmentally delayed and that there is a hierarchy of progression with normally developing children faster in total movement time than children who are clumsy, intellectually disabled or with Down syndrome. Finally, similarities were found in the spatial accuracy measure which showed that none of these children differed from each other, in meeting the spatial-accuracy requirements of the movement task.

Conclusion

Both similarities and differences in patterns of motor development have been found among groups of clumsy, intellectually disabled and Down syndrome children, such results indicate that adapted motor programmes for similarly impaired children should include activities which generally enhance their current level of development while specifically addressing some of the problems which are unique to their particular category of impairment. Recommendations to develop well-designed developmental intervention programmes will be discussed briefly in the next section.

RECOMMENDATIONS FOR ADAPTED MOTOR PROGRAMMES FOR CHILDREN WHO ARE CLUMSY, INTELLECTUALLY DISABLED AND WITH DOWN SYNDROME

General guidelines for implementing adapted motor programmes are discussed first, before presenting guidelines for more specific intervention.

General guidelines for adapted motor programmes

A priority in designing an adapted motor programme is to use motor assessment tests which are sufficiently diagnostic to

Table 7.2 Activity guidelines based on the hierarchy of movement behaviour and the behavioural model

Hierarchy of movement behaviour	*Control levels adapted from the neurobehavioural model*	*Levels for programming and specific activity guidelines*
	Basic control processes	*Level 1 (sensory-neurological)*
Reflexes Intertask movements	Control over primitive reflexes and initial stability control	*Sensory motor activities, emphasis on vestibular, kinaesthetic, tactile and visual modalities. *Generalized movement experiences using total body movements combined with sensory input.
	Sensory systems	*Specific Activity Guidelines* +Activities which incorporate spinning, rocking, sliding and those that increase general body awareness by providing extra resistance to joints and muscles through hanging, climbing, bouncing etc.
	Intermediate control processes	*Level 2 (integrative-perceptual)*
Intratask movements	Postural control	*Extension of sensory motor activities. *Extension of balance activities. *Interlimb coordination activities.

Intratask movements *contd*	Interlimb control Hand/foot–eye coordination Sensory integration	*Hand/foot–eye coordination activities. *Specific Activity Guidelines* +Play equipment to increase sensory motor input e.g., swings, ropes, slides. +Encourage more advanced balance activities on large equipment, and by use of stilts and rocker boards. +Increase interlimb and hand/foot–eye coordination by simple games, dance.
	Advanced control processes	*Level 3 (motor learning-control)*
Movement skills	Ability to process more relevant sensory information; can cope with faster input Ability to control spatial-temporal and force aspects of complex movements and sport and recreational skills	*Advanced sensory motor, postural control and coordination activities *Advanced ability to coordinate limbs and control body to meet difficult spatial-temporal demands. *Control of lengthy movement sequences. *Specific Activity Guidelines* +Improve the above through activities such as aerobics, dancing, gymnastics movement sequences.

*Variety in adapted motor programmes is important.

enable appropriate activities to be devised for motor impaired children, and with the scope to give information about the particular needs of each child. A further requirement of the diagnostic test is that it is ecologically valid in that the tasks used in the test parallel normal movement situations. For example, if the child is required to catch a ball, is it thrown at sufficient speed and from a distance which would replicate a situation in children's games at this age. Finally, it is important that the test is based on a comprehensive model of motor development.

Another important consideration in designing and implementing an adapted motor programme is that the people conducting the programme have a thorough knowledge of normally developing children's motor performance, fundamental movement patterns and the motor learning and control processes that underlie their movement behaviour. If the person designing the adapted motor programme does not have this knowledge, then the programme is unlikely to improve the skills of motor impaired children, because the activities will not be at the appropriate developmental level, or they will not be suitable for remediation of the specific movement problems of particular groups of motor impaired children.

The results from the three measures of movement behaviour which were used in this book meet the first two criteria, because they provide diagnostic information and the tasks are based on knowledge of children's movement behaviour (the only proviso being that the ball throw and catching tasks in the BOT-S are probably too simple to provide useful information about how children use these skills in games). It is proposed, therefore, that the results from the three measures of movement behaviour used in this book provide a suitable basis for framing guidelines for the implementation of adapted motor programmes designed to improve the behavioural functioning of the different categories of motor impaired children, who were studied here.

Specific guidelines, derived from the studies in this book, will be discussed in the next two sections which deal with adapted motor programmes aimed at improving the motor skills of motor impaired children, in early and middle childhood. These guidelines are presented in a summary form in Table 7.2, which is based on the hierarchy of movement behaviour and the basic, intermediate and advanced processes that affect motor development, which were outlined in Chapter 1. It also provides some programming ideas for each of the three phases of motor development.

Specific guidelines for adapted programmes for motor impaired children in early childhood

The results from the studies of the three measures of movement behaviour have revealed that the younger age group of motor impaired children have many deficits in basic control processes that affect their motor development, they are, therefore, still in the first phase of motor control. They also showed that their intermediate control processes are not well developed because they had poorer balance skills and bilateral coordination than their normally developing peers. For these reasons an adapted motor programme for motor impaired children (aged 4–7 years) should aim to enhance sensory motor functioning and, specifically to emphasize vestibular and proprioceptive information, which should improve balance and general body awareness (sensory–motor activities). Such activities appear to be particularly important for children who are clumsy or have Down syndrome, as many of them appear to have specific balance deficits at this age.

The apparent immaturity of the younger motor impaired children, in comparison with normally developing children, in the locomotor skills of walking, running and jumping, would indicate that practice in many variations of these skills should be incorporated in adapted motor programmes (Level 2 in the activities section). Activities which emphasize lower limb proprioception and control are particularly important for children with Down syndrome who appear to have a specific problem in controlling their lower limbs in locomotor patterns.

The younger motor impaired children as a group also had immature levels in throwing and catching as well as poorer performance in these skills, in comparison with their normal peers. These findings support claims in the literature that the ability, particularly of the children who were intellectually disabled or with Down syndrome, to respond to visual–spatial information is lower than their normally developing peers. Motor impaired children, therefore, should be given additional activities which encourage them to make visual–spatial responses, such as reacting to and controllng moving objects (Level 2 hand–eye coordination, in the activities section).

In summary, the younger motor impaired children who participated in the studies in this book showed deficits in basic body control in controlling the action of their limbs and in controlling their body while interacting with external objects.

Specific guidelines for adapted motor programmes for motor impaired children in middle childhood

Results from the studies in this book indicated that by middle childhood there were differences in movement behaviour among the older clumsy children, as their performance and the maturity of their fundamental movement patterns was consistently higher than their other motor impaired peers. This trend was not apparent in the younger clumsy children when their movement behaviour was compared with their motor impaired peers.

The fact that older clumsy children had higher performance scores than their motor impaired peers, may be related to their superior cognitive ability, which enables them to acquire greater control of their movements. As a result of increased cognitive ability they may be able to process and respond to movement information more efficiently than the children with intellectual disability or Down syndrome. This interpretation, although consistent with the behavioural perspective that was proposed in this book, can only be verified by further research. Children with intellectual disability and Down syndrome were not as competent in motor skills, however, as normally developing children of the same age. The findings from the present studies indicate that apart from a motor programme suitable for normally developing children, at a similar movement skill level, clumsy children should be given extra practice in interlimb coordination and general motor skills (Levels 2 and 3 activities, in the next section).

From the results of the studies it is apparent that children who are intellectually disabled, and especially children with Down syndrome, have continuing problems in controlling their movements. These problems limit their ability to adapt to the changing environment. In addition, these children demonstrated less capacity to modify the spatial–temporal characteristics of their movements. As a result they have a less varied repertoire of movement skills. For these reasons they may still need a programme which aims to enhance their sensory–motor and perceptual–motor development (Levels 1 and 2 activities, in the next section).

The difference between the early childhood activities, and those suitable for the older children with intellectual disability or Down syndrome children of the same age and with similar movement behaviour, is that they should be appropriate for the chronological age of these older children. For example, kinaesthesis, proprioception and body awareness may be enhanced by a fitness programme, weight training or simple games and dance. To ensure variety and to enhance their motor development, practice should also be given in many relatively complex motor skills such as those in gymnastics to facilitate learning and to develop better voluntary control of movement. In addition, it would appear that emphasis should be given to activities that encourage hand–eye coordination in intellectually disabled, as well as clumsy children because their manipulative skills were at a lower level of development than their locomotor skills.

ACTIVITIES SUITABLE FOR SENSORY-MOTOR, PERCEPTUAL-MOTOR AND COGNITIVE-MOTOR DEVELOPMENT

This section provides examples of activities which can be used both in developmental and adapted motor programmes.

To aid professionals in their programming, motor development was conceptualized in this book as being divided into three phases. First, children gain basic control over their body. Once this has been achieved it is then possible for children to control their body in different environmental situations, followed by control over the spatial–temporal, force and accuracy components of complex skills. The way in which children developed these three phases of motor control can be conceptualized as sensory-motor (first phase), perceptual-motor (second phase) and cognitive-motor (third phase) phases of development. These levels of motor control can be correlated with the levels of motor development that children exhibit in their fundamental movement patterns which in turn influences the choice of activity ideas, as summarized next.

1. Children who have most of their fundamental movement patterns at level 1 and some at level 2 will benefit from sensory-motor activities which emphasize vestibular, kinaesthetic, tactile and visual modalities. These children are still utilizing sensory feedback to learn about their environment and to acquire basic control of movement. Gross motor activities to enhance children's motor development at this level include spinning, rocking, sliding and bouncing activities to increase vestibular awareness, and hanging, climbing and weight-bearing activities to provide extra resistance to joints and muscles in order to increase kinaesthetic input, and so improve general body awareness.
2. Children who have most of their movement patterns between levels 2 and 3 will benefit from perceptual-motor activities that involve integrative-perceptual processes which require them to practise movements that place greater demands on sensory integration, balance and interlimb control. Activities which incorporate some of these requirements can be achieved by the type of equipment children use in their play or that is provided for them. Examples of play equipment to encourage perceptual-motor development would include swings, slippery slides and ropes, more advanced balance activities on large equipment and on small equipment such as stilts, rocker boards and bicycles. Interlimb control can be improved by encouraging children to practise their locomotor and manipulative fundamental movement patterns in a variety of play, games and in simple movement sequences, games and dance.
3. Children who have movement patterns at levels 3 and 4 will also benefit from perceptual-motor activities because they have more advanced control over their stability, interlimb coordination and better control over the spatial-temporal, force and accuracy components of complex movements. Specific activities would include traditional childhood games such as hopscotch, rope skipping and games with balls. In addition, they would benefit from activities such as aerobics and from learning dance, gymnastics, sport and recreational skills.

It should be noted that before starting any of these activities with motor impaired children precautions must be taken, depending on the severity of their condition. For example, children who are clumsy often have difficulty controlling the force of their movements, and many of them have have poor balance and fall easily. Children with Down syndrome not only have these problems, but many of them also have major physical problems. One of these problems is atlanto-axial instability, which means any flexion such as when the head is flexed in a forward roll, or pressure is applied to the neck or the head is in extreme extension, is likely to cause subluxation in this neck joint. Another major consideration before conducting a programme for children with Down syndrome is that many of them have cardiac abnormalities and in some this condition cannot be medically corrected, so intense physical activity is not recommended.

General sensory-motor activities

The majority of the activities listed below under general sensory-motor activities, are suitable for very young or developmentally delayed children. They are based on movement activities which stimulate the tactile, kinaesthetic, vestibular and visual sensory systems.

- Rolling in all directions on a mat or soft surface
- Activities which incorporate going through, under or over equipment
- Rolling down an incline
- Spinning on a scooter board
- Propelling or pulling oneself along on a scooter board
- Creeping, or belly crawling, across a mat or slippery surface
- Imitating other people's postures while sitting and standing
- Mimicking the way various animals walk
- Rolling in barrels
- Child rolled up in a rug or mat then unrolled
- Child swung backwards and forwards, while supported in a rug
- Walk and then jump into hoops placed on the floor in a variety of patterns
- Kick, hit or push a large, light, inflated ball with various body parts

- Play a game solving body puzzles using different placements of symbols of the body
- Play with a balloon or large, light beach ball
- Blowing, chasing and trying to catch bubbles
- Follow a line maze taped or drawn on the floor
- Play musical and imitation movement games
- Child being rocked while leaning back against an adult who is sitting on the floor
- Child being rocked and moved in the arms of an adult dancing to different rhythms

Advanced sensory-motor activities

- Parachute games
  (a) holding onto edge of parachute and walking around clockwise and anticlockwise
  (b) running around and changing direction on an auditory signal
  (c) make waves with the parachute with some children stamping on the waves
  (d) float parachute up in the air and some children run underneath
- Climbing and swinging on large equipment
- Walking over swinging bridges
- Crawling, walking, running around on a trampoline
- Produce different patterns of movement on a rebounder, such as a star jumping and stretching tall etc.

Vestibular activities

- Swing and spin on swings or in tyre seats
- Slide down an inclined board or slippery slide, feet first and head first
- Roll down an incline in tyre tubes roped together
- Crawl, walk, run, jump over a swinging bridge with eyes open, then with eyes shut
- Ride prone on scooter board, manoeuvring it between obstacles

Activities to improve strength and body awareness

These activities are also suitable for children with low muscle tone, and for improving kinaesthetic awareness.

Upper limbs and trunk

- Wheelbarrow walks
- Crab walk
- Hanging from an overhead bar a rope or horizontal ladder
- Climbing activities on a scrambling net, ladder ropes and poles
- Measuring worm; with hands stationary, walk feet to hands, then keep feet stationary and walk hands to feet
- Frog hop; from squat position leap forward to place hands on floor, then the feet
- Seal walk; lie flat on floor, push upper body off floor by the arms and drag lower limbs along the ground.

Lower limbs

- Jump imitating different types of animals, e.g., kangaroo, cat, frog
- Jump as far, as high and in as many different ways as you can
- Sequence of jumps on the tyre tube or a trampoline
- Jump off different heights
- Jump into a series of hoops
- Jump sideways over a line and back again
- Leap from one foot onto the other
- Jump over a rope being moved in a 'snake' like pattern

General coordination and body awareness

- *Find out how large your body parts are:* (1) Move your hands down the length of your arm, where does it start and where does it stop? Repeat using leg. (2) Place two hands around your waist, how big is it? How can you move at the waist Try bending forward, sidewards, backwards, twist around at the waist. Compare the size of two parts of the body, e.g. arm/leg, waist/shoulders, ankle/wrist, kneel/elbow etc.

- *Touch* ear to shoulder, shoulder to knee, nose to knee, elbow to thigh, knee to ankle, toe to knee, toe to chin
- *Make body prints* in the sand with front, back, side, elbow, knee, foot and hand
- *Body awareness rhyme*:

  'Hands on your shoulders
  Hands on your knees
  Hands behind you
  If you please.

  Touch your tummy,
  Now your toes
  Now your head
  Now your nose.

  Hands up high in the air
  Now down to your side
  Then touch your hair.

  Hands up high as before
  Now clap your hands, 1,2,3,4,
  And now if you please
  Sit on the floor'.

- Children play '*Simon Says*', while lying on their backs. Lift one leg, hold it, lower it. Repeat using the other leg. Move one leg out to the side along the floor, bring it back. Repeat using the other leg. Lift one leg, cross it over the other leg, touch the floor if possible. Repeat using the other leg. Do similar actions with the arms .
- Children play '*Back to Back*'. Each child stands 'back to back' with another child. One child is without a partner. This child calls out the next command e.g. 'face to face' or 'side to side' or 'back to back'. On this command all children must change partners with the extra player also seeking a partner. Variations: everyone can hop, skip, jump, walk like an elephant etc. until the command is given.
- Children play 'Where can you Bend'? Encourage the children to experiment with moving the following joints in as many ways as possible – jaws, neck, shoulders, elbows and wrists.

- *Move and sing*:
  Caterpillar crawling around
  Where green and juicy leaves are found
  Soon a silk cocoon you'll spin
  Winding threads 'til you're within
  When spring comes bye and bye
  Flutter out a butterfly

  and

- Jack in the box is out of sight
  When the cover is fastened tight
  Lift the lock and up it goes
  Jack in the box with his hopping toes.

Perceptual-motor activities

In the perceptual-motor phase, children have sufficient knowledge and experience in movement situations to have developed relatively mature postural stability and body awareness. As well as enhancing these two areas of development, emphasis should now be placed on concepts such as laterality and directionality, spatial awareness of one's own body in relation to external objects, visual–spatial awareness enabling judgements to be made about speed and direction of moving objects and accurate manipulation of tools and objects.

Additionally, there should be opportunities to practise the fundamental movement patterns and extension of these patterns so that children achieve greater control of their limbs and postural stability, as well as early control of the visual–spatial parameters of movement. For this reason varieties of activities and games should include variations of the fundamental movement patterns and extension of these patterns, such as skipping and galloping, running and dodging, jumping over and off different heights, and experimenting with projecting and intercepting many types of moving objects.

Postural stability

Static balance

- Balance on both feet bend trunk to one side and then the other

- Balance on both feet with eyes shut
- Balance on one foot, then the other
- Stand on tiptoes with feet together
- Stand on heels with feet together
- Balance on different body parts, and at different levels
- Turn around while balancing on one foot
- Stand on one leg and swing the other
- Make a V-shape of your body
- Stand on both feet and twist, turn and make circles with the upper body
- Stand on a sheet of newspaper, then fold it in half, keep repeating this process until the paper is so small that maintaining balance becomes difficult

Dynamic balance

- Walk forward, backward, sideways on the jouncing board (a springy plank of wood)
- Jump on both feet along the jouncing board
- Hop on either foot along the jouncing board
- Walk along balance board and step over obstacles such as ropes, hoops or blocks
- Walk along balance board and step between bean bags
- Walk along balance board, pick up an object, turn and hop back
- Walk up and down an inclined balance board
- Walk along balance board with bean bag on head
- Walk on 'coffee can' stilts
- Explore lying, sitting on a large barrel
- Walk around hoop

Locomotor activities

- *Duck walk*; waddle forward in crouch position, hold hands flat behind back, fingers pointing away fron the body to form a duck's tail.
- *Bear walk*; walk on hands and feet keeping the legs and arm straight.
- *Ostrich walk*; bend forward at the waist and grasp ankles, keep knees stiff and walk forward stretching the neck in and out.

- *Kangaroo hop*; crouch, fingers touching the floor between the knees, then jump up and forward, bodies stretched, then land in a crouched position.
- *Crab walk*; squat reach backwards, place hands flat on the floor behind the hips (without sitting down). Raise pelvis as high as possible, then move backwards and forwards in this position and try to keep head, neck and trunk parallel to the floor.
- *Bunny hop*; raise hands to the side of the head, squat on heels, hop on both feet, wiggle 'ears' as you hop.
- *Crane dance*; stand and raise one leg off the floor, keep knees straight, raise both arms to the side at shoulder height, hop on one foot turning to the left in a circle and then turn to the right, then repeat on the other leg.
- *Troll walk*; children are angry trolls; they walk by raising their knees high and stamping their feet. Trunks are bent forward and their arms are held stiffly, because they are so angry. Then they begin to feel happier so they stamp less and their arms swing freely, finally their bodies are straight and their arms are relaxed.
- *Tightrope walker*; children pretend to be a tightrope walker at the circus. Encourage then to hold out their pole and walk slowly in a straight line, pretending to lose and regain balance.
- Run in zig zags and around an obstacle course.
- Play the following games:

Follow the leader: children must follow the movements of the leader, for example, the leader may stop suddenly, crouch, jump sideways, walk on all fours etc.

Space ship game (running): children stand in free formation, an object such as a hoop is chosen to represent the earth. The children are space ships and on the countdown, 5,4,3,2,1. BLAST OFF the space ships quickly gather speed and go into orbit around the earth. After one or more orbits the space ships return and 'splash down' in the same area from where they blasted off. Repeat with variations such as rockets going out of control and twisting and tumbling in orbit.

Flowers in the wind (movement skill running and dodging): two lines of children facing each other. One line of children is designated as flowers the other as the wind. The flowers decide which particular flower they will be and then they advance towards the wind. While the 'flowers' are advancing the 'wind' tries to guess what kind of flower they have selected. 'Flowers' answer yes or no as they walk forward slowly. When the right flower is named the 'wind' chases the 'flowers' back to the starting line. All persons tagged join the wind group. The game is continued until all persons are caught. OR the groups can alternate roles.

Green light, red light (to enhance starting and stopping skills and to enhance listening skills): the group lines up at one end of a designated area. One player 'IT' stands at least 10 m away with his/her back to the group. The game begins with 'IT' calling 'green light'. When this is heard the other children begin to move forward. Then 'IT' calls 'red light' and turns quickly to face the children. 'IT' calls the name of any children who have not completely stopped. These children must return to the starting line and start again. The first child to cross the line where 'IT' is standing becomes the next 'IT'.

The big giant (running and dodging): one child (the big giant) lives in a 'paddock' in the centre of a designated area. On one side of the area are the other children, who want to cross the paddock to get to the forest on the other side. The giant shouts 'Who's afraid of the big strong giant?' The children answer, 'No one' and try to run across the paddock to the forest without being caught by the giant, who is not allowed to leave the 'paddock'. Whoever is caught first becomes the next giant.

Crows and cranes (running, dodging, pivoting, starting and stopping): two lines of children face each other about four metres apart. One line comprises the group called the crows the other group is called the cranes. On a signal the two groups move towards each other. The teacher then calls either 'crows' or 'cranes', if the crows are called they chase the cranes back to the nest and the children who are caught become crows and vice versa.

Hand–eye, body–eye coordination activities

- Use either cardboard rolls or hands to keep a balloon or light beach ball in the air
- Use a cardboard roll to hit a balloon to another person
- Hit the balloon into the air with your head
- Catch a bean bag or nerf ball thrown in the air
- Throw a bean bag, sock ball or nerf ball into a large container
- Throw an object at a clown target
- Roll a hoop forward, backward or in a straight line, run alongside and try to catch it
- Roll a hoop to a partner on a balance board
- Dodge a soft ball thrown at you
- Bounce a ball into a hoop with both hands, then one hand
- Catch a large ball thrown at different speeds and in different directions
- Play catching with a partner, first bouncing, then throwing to one another
- Shoot for baskets placed at an appropriate height

Spatial awareness activities

- Chant or sing and move to:

  I can climb so very high
  I can almost reach the sky
  I can climb most anything
  I'm a puppet on a string.

- Outline the children's bodies on a sheet of newsprint while they are lying on their backs. Have the children cut out their bodies, colour them, dress them, compare sizes, hang up their bodies.
- Children in free space, ask them to make themselves as small as possible, e.g., like a small ball; then have the children make themselves as tall or as wide as possible, make them aware of the fact that as they get bigger or wider they take up more space.
- Ask the children to take a partner and then spread out. One child is to shut his/her eyes while the other child gives directions on how to reach the treasure, e.g., ten steps forwards, one jump sideways, two steps backwards.

- Walk through a maze of chairs, tables or some other suitable objects; step over, crawl under and step on objects, then try the maze while blindfolded
- Crawl through tunnels with eyes open and shut
- Solve complex footprint, handprint puzzles
- Hide in a small place
- Children hold their hands together in front of their bodies, then step their feet over their hands and back again
- Working with a partner and using either ropes and hoops, pretend to be a worm crawling under the obstacle
- Place ropes on the floor in various patterns and geometric shapes, e.g., wavy lines, zig zag lines, circles, squares and triangles; have the children walk along or around the shapes
- Visually remember an obstacle course then negotiate it blindfolded.

Body awareness, (laterality, unilateral, bilateral and contralateral movement activities)

- For laterality and bilateral awareness chant or sing Looby Loo:

  Here we dance looby loo
  Here we dance looby light
  Here we dance lobby loo
  All on a Saturday night

  Then

  I put my right hand in
  I take my right hand out
  I give my right hand a shake, shake, shake
  And turn myself about
  I put my left hand in etc.
  I put my right foot in etc.
  I put my left foot in etc.
  I put my head way in etc.
  I put my whole self in etc.

- Tell the children about centipedes and how when they are touched they curl up into a tight ball. Children then roll about like centipedes in all directions without bumping each other; on a command they assume a log rolling position.

- Children pretend to be puppets, they stiffly move their legs or arms, or both, after their partner touches the limbs to be moved. Extend this activity so that when the children are touched on the legs they must walk in a stiff puppet walk etc.
- Practise transferring weight from one body part to another, then onto different sides of the body, an arm and leg on opposite sides, then on the same side.
- Join hands with a partner and spin one another around as fast as possible.
- Try to jump on your own shadow, or on another person's shadow.

Rhythm

- Play hot and cold; an object is hidden anywhere in the room and a child tries to find it by listening to the loudness or softness of the clapping of the other children. The clapping should become louder as the child gets closer to the object.
- Adult claps rhythmic patterns and the children move about in time with the beat.
- Children listen with eyes shut to a clapped rhythm and then they must repeat it and move to it.
- A trip to the zoo; use various instruments to represent different animals, when the children hear the different sounds they move like the animal that the sound represents, e.g., a triangle for a bird, rhythmic sticks for galloping horses.
- Play singing and moving games like looby loo, here we go round the mulberry bush.

Relaxation

- Be a balloon, feel very light, gradually float up off the ground, then float slowly back to the ground.
- Be an ice block, big and round, and when the sun shines melt to the ground.
- Lie in a sleep position and relax completely from toes to head.

- 'Windy weather' Like a leaf or a feather, in the windy, windy, weather, we will whirl and twirl around and all sink down together.
- Children to be 'rag dolls' or 'floppy teddy bears', first standing, then lying down. Call out arm, leg, back, head etc. These body parts must be moved like a 'rag doll' or a 'floppy teddy bear'.

Cognitive-motor activities

The third phase of motor development is shown in the acquisition of more complex movement skills, which involve processing relevant external environmental information, as well as controlling the spatial–temporal, force and accuracy components of the response. These processes are used by children in their games, sport and recreational activities. For example, in order to intercept a moving ball children need to process complex visual information while at the same time achieving precise body control. Once children have attained this level of development they are ready for more traditional movement skills such as gymnastics, dancing and sport, but they may still be challenged by more complex childhood games such as those listed below. For example:

- Hopscotch
- Elastics
- Rope skipping
- Many of the low competitive playground ball games, such as corners, sevens, hand tennis etc.
- Children are ready to participate in modified sports activities.
- Children are ready to learn simple gymnastics skills (see Primary School Syllabus)
- Children are ready to learn folk and other forms of dancing (see Primary School Syllabus)

IMPLICATIONS OF THE PRESENT STUDIES FOR MOTOR DEVLEOPMENT

The behavioural model developed for this book has provided a valuable framework for examining movement behaviour in motor impaired children. By classifying movement behaviour in terms of sensory-neurological, integrative-perceptual and motor learning-control processes, it has enabled the synthesis of information in seemingly separate areas, the development of sensory motor and perceptual-motor skills and cognitive control of movement. It has also enabled a more comprehensive examination of the movement behaviour of motor impaired children than when only one aspect of movement is studied.

In applying this perspective to motor development, it was found that younger motor impaired groups of children have lower levels of motor development than groups of older motor impaired children, as is the case in the normally developing children. Each one of the measures used to study the motor impaired children, however, produced separate patterns of results which in some instances suggest that motor impaired children are developmentally delayed, whereas in others they indicate that these children are developmentally different. For instance, over the three measures used in this book to study movement behaviour, none of the motor impaired children demonstrated a pattern of progression similar to that of normally developing children, and patterns of difference among the groups were not consistent. These findings, therefore, do not support the concept that delay characterizes the motor impairment of these children. In addition, the increased rate of change in movement behaviour across the groups of younger and older clumsy children, in comparison with other groups of motor impaired children, is supported by the findings of the motor control studies. The apparent acceleration in motor development is probably due to superior cognitive ability. This enables clumsy children to control their movements more easily and may compensate for deficits in some of the basic and intermediate processes that affect their movement behaviour.

The motor control measures identified some of the underlying cognitive processes that may help explain some of the differences in movement behaviour, observed by many researchers of motor development of motor impaired children. In particular, this book has provided some preliminary evidence that the slow movements of children with intellectual disability or Down syndrome have been shown to be caused by differences in motor control processes. The slow response of intellectually disabled children may make it difficult for them to respond quickly to new movement situations. Conversely, the movement time results of the children with Down syndrome suggest that even though they can organize a movement response relatively quickly, they are slower than their intellectually disabled peers in actually moving their limbs to complete a movement task. Some of this slowness in movement may be related to their low muscle tone as well as to biological and integrative deficits in the formulation and the timing and force parameters of movement.

Of all the measures which were derived from the behavioural perspective adopted in this book, the motor control measures appear to have the best prospect of providing insights into the observable differences in movement behaviour in motor impaired children. It is claimed, therefore, that a greater knowledge of how children acquire motor control is essential, not only for our understanding of motor development, but also for the design and implementation of more effective motor programmes. At present there is little knowledge about how children control their movements because, until recently, there had been a lack of research in this area of motor development.

Finally, the preliminary evidence from the studies in this book supports the notion that children, whether they are normally developing or motor impaired, do not attain similar levels in all the areas of motor development. This finding supports the position proposed by theorists in the area of cognitive development. The results from the studies in this book, however, highlight a more general developmental issue. This issue encompasses the heterogeneous aspects of development and the scope for individual differences, irrespective of the area of development or the category of impairment. The uniformity implied by terms such as 'developmental delay', in the final analysis, may prove more apparent than real.

Appendix A
Details of children participating in the study and the tests and procedures used

DETAILS OF THE CHILDREN WHO PARTICIPATED IN THE STUDIES

Preliminary screening of motor impaired children

The data on motor impaired children that are reported in the studies in this book were collected from samples of children who were referred to the Child Motor Performance Centre (Department of Human Movement Studies, University of Queensland, Brisbane, Australia), because of suspected movement problems. The children were aged between 4 and 11 years of age and the majority of them could be classified as clumsy, intellectually disabled or with Down syndrome.

All children were screened on the first five subtests of the Bruininks–Oseretsky Test of Motor Proficiency (BOT-S). A review of the literature had revealed that the first four subtests incorporated items that were the most sensitive measures of children's total motor performance scores (e.g. Broadhead and Bruininks, 1983a; Haubenstricker *et al.*, 1981). Additionally, the subtest measuring ball skills was included in this abbreviated screening test because it assessed gross motor skills commonly required in children's games.

The next section of this Appendix outlines information about the four different categories of children who participated in the studies, and the rationale for the selection of age groupings.

Characteristics of the children studied

Groups, drawn from four categories of children, participated in the series of studies. The first two categories comprised children who attended normal schools and had normal motor skills, and clumsy children who attended normal schools but had motor problems. The other two categories comprised motor impaired intellectually disabled children. One category included children with idiopathic intellectual disability, in the mild to moderate range of severity. The other category, children with Down syndrome, were similarly intellectually impaired. None of these children who comprised the clumsy, intellectually disabled or Down syndrome categories had been diagnosed as having cerebral palsy or any other neuromotor disease.

The clumsy children were chosen on the basis that their scores were at least one year lower than the age norm on the adapted version of the Bruininks–Oseretsky Motor Performance Test used in this project. The clumsy children were considered a comparison group for the other motor impaired children who had motor and intellectual impairment. All the clumsy children had been referred by parents, therapists, teachers or doctors to the clinic.

The intellectually disabled children were selected because they represented a population with known motor impairment. They were of particular interest as traditionally they have been considered developmentally delayed. Children with Down syndrome, because of their specific chromosomal abnormality and its neurological and physical implications, are increasingly considered different in their development from their normal and intellectually disabled peers.

As stated, the intellectually disabled and Down syndrome group of children who participated in the studies fell within the mild to moderate range of intellectual handicap. Children with moderate retardation have IQ scores on intelligence tests of 35–40 to 50–55 and those with IQ scores between 50–55 and

70, are regarded as having mild retardation (Kirk and Gallagher, 1986). The authors were unable to obtain scores on intelligence tests for all the children, but on the basis of their school placement, and advice from guidance personnel and psychologists monitoring the children's progress, it could be assumed that all children were within the mild to moderate categories of intellectual disabilities. For example, all but three attended Special Schools. One criterion for placement in a Special School is that children have an intellectual disability of mild to moderate severity. Evidence from the Schonell Centre, University of Queensland, indicated that the three children with Down syndrome who attended regular schools were also in the mild to moderate categories. Moreover, all children in the two intellectually disabled groups were at least one year below the age norms on the adaptation of the Bruininks–Oseretsky Test of Motor Proficiency.

Ages of children who participated in the studies

In order to examine age-related changes in movement behaviour, all the children who participated in the studies could be allocated to two groups, designated the early and middle childhood groups. The age ranges were 4–7 years (approximately) for the younger or early childhood group, and 8–11 years (approximately), for the older or middle childhood group. The exact ages are reported in each study. The majority of reviewed studies dealing with motor impaired children have used similar age groupings. Furthermore, these age groupings approximate known brain growth spurts.

THE BRUININKS–OSERETSKY TEST OF MOTOR PROFICIENCY

The Bruininks–Oseretsky Test of Motor Proficiency (BOT) was adapted by Bruininks (1978) from the Oseretsky Test of Motor Proficiency. Approximately 40% of items were retained from the original version devised by Oseretsky and the remainder are new items (Broadhead and Bruininks, 1982). The BOT is designed to measure motor proficiency in children aged 4 years 6 months to 14 years 6 months of age. The full test consists of eight subtests with 46 separate items and it takes about one hour to administer. Raw scores are converted into a standardized composite score for gross motor skills, for fine motor skills and for the total battery. The Short Form comprises 14 items from the Complete Battery, divided into gross motor, gross and fine motor and fine motor areas. Normative data from the full version and the Short Form of the BOT includes standard scores for each age group (at six monthly intervals), percentile ranks, stanines and age equivalents, for each of the eight subtests (Bruininks, 1978).

Bruininks (1978) stated that a comprehensive literature review of factors affecting motor performance revealed several qualitatively different aspects of gross and fine motor development, which were used as a guide in developing items that comprised the test. In gross motor ability he included items that measured gross motor speed, static balance, dynamic balance, coordinated movements and strength. Gross and fine motor abilities were measured by items that required the coordination of visual input with arm and hand movements. Fine motor abilities were measured by response speed to a moving target, visual motor control or eye–hand coordination and upper limb speed and precision.

In the final standardization sample for the BOT there were 756 children aged between 4 years 6 months to 14 years 6 months of age. Each age group was divided into boys and girls with approximately equal numbers, except for the 13 years 6 months to 14 years 6 months old group, which consisted of 23 boys and only 12 girls. The maximum number of children in an age grouping was 56 and the lowest number was 12 children. Attempts were also made to keep the factors race and community size in proportion with those reported by the 1970 US census.

Bruininks (1978) claimed his test was valid, reliable and met test–retest reliability criteria. His test–retest reliability study, however, was conducted on only 63 normally developing second grade children (mean age, 8 years 2 months) and 63 sixth grade children (mean age, 12 years 2 months). As well as standardizing and validating the subtests on normally developing subjects, Bruininks conducted three further studies to determine if intellectually disabled and learning disabled subjects scored lower than normal peers on the test battery.

Subsequent studies by Bruininks and other researchers, since the publication of the test in 1978, have re-analysed the original data and resulted in the following findings.

1. When the data are grouped into three different age categories (under 5 years, 5–9 years, and over 9 years), general motor abilities can be defined using factor analytical techniques. The general motor abilities identified from data on the full version of the BOT were balance, strength and bilateral coordination (Krus, Bruininks and Robertson, 1981).
2. When the short form of the BOT-S was re-analysed using the original data, but dividing it into four groups (boys and girls, aged 4 years 5 months to 9 years 5 months and 9 years 6 months to 14 years 5 months), four subtests of the gross motor component were shown to contribute most to the change in motor performance scores with increased age. These four subtests were running speed and agility, balance, bilateral coordination and strength (Broadhead and Bruininks, 1983a).
3. When the data of the BOT-S were re-analysed, with boys and girls in yearly age groups, it was found that most of the tests did not distinguish between boys and girls at each age level. The exceptions were running speed and agility, and strength. The two balance tests also distinguished between only half the age categories for boys whereas upper limb speed and dexterity distinguished between half the girl's age categories (Broadhead and Bruininks, 1983b).
4. A re-analysis of the raw data on all of the subtests of the BOT-S (by boys and girls and using 10 age groups of yearly intervals) revealed that there was a significant difference in performance on all the items in the subtests, at all ages for the boys and in 13 of the 14 items for the girls. There was also evidence of increasing differentiation between motor abilities at increased age. Boys were superior in gross motor performance in the subtests of running speed and agility, and strength (as measured by the standing broad jump). Whereas, girls were superior in the balance and coordination subtests. In fine motor abilities boys were better at the response speed subtest and girls were better at the upper limb speed and dexterity subtest (Broadhead and Bruininks, 1982).
5. Analysis of the BOT-S raw data revealed that there was rapid improvement in motor performance in children between 5 and 11 years of age with a subsequent levelling off in performance in older children (Broadhead and Bruininks, 1982).

USE OF THE BOT ON EXCEPTIONAL CHILDREN

Bruininks (1978) reported that the BOT discriminated between normal, learning disabled and mildly and moderately intellectually disabled children. Several other studies have used the BOT on exceptional populations, and these will be reported next.

A study by Haubenstricker *et al.* (1981) tested the sensitivity of the BOT as a screening device for children with suspected motor problems, referred to a Remedial Motor Clinic. The subjects were 62 boys, aged between 6 and 10 years. The mean age of the remedial motor group was 7 years 9 months ($n=31$), and the mean age of the children with normal motor skills was 8 years 1 month (n=31). All the children attended regular schools (six of the remedial group attended special education classes for a few hours a day). None of the children had been diagnosed as physically impaired at the time of testing.

Haubenstricker *et al.* (1981) stated that although the BOT distinguished between normal and mildly to moderately intellectually handicapped children, no study had been undertaken to see whether the test would discriminate between normal children and those with suspected coordination problems i.e., clumsy children). Their results, demonstrated that the BOT did discriminate between these two groups of children, since the normally developing boys attained significantly higher scores than the boys with coordination problems, on the gross motor composite (subtests: running speed and agility, balance, bilateral coordination and strength), the gross and fine motor battery and the fine motor battery.

In another study children with mild learning disabilities were administered the full version of the BOT and their scores were compared with data from matched subjects who participated in the original BOT project (Bruininks and Bruininks, 1977). The children in this study($n=5$ in each category) were aged from 6 to 13 years (mean age, 9 years 3 months). The results were similar to those reported in the Bruininks–Oseretsky Test Manual (1978). Normally developing children had significantly better overall motor performance than learning disabled children on all tasks except response speed. The learning disabled children were shown to have major problems in balance skills, bilateral coordination and visual–motor coordination.

The evidence then, from both studies (Bruininks *et al.*, 1977; Haubenstricker *et al.*, 1981), suggests that specific motor dysfunction occurs in learning disabled and clumsy children.

The two preceding studies used the full version of the BOT on normally developing and special populations, however, the next two studies to be reported used the BOT-S. The first study was by Roswal (1983), who used the BOT-S to determine the pre- and post-programme effects of a play programme on the motor development of mildly intellectually disabled children (n = 27), aged between 9 and 12 years. The Short Form of the test was selected because Roswal considered it easy to administer and the children enjoyed participating in the test. Roswal's study confirmed that the BOT-S is an appropriate test for handicapped children in this age range.

A second study using the BOT-S was conducted on 49 normal and 18 mildly and moderately intellectually disabled children, aged 5 to 12 years (Broadhead and Church, 1982). The twofold purpose of the study was to ascertain, first the usefulness of the BOT-S to determine physical education placement for mildly to moderately intellectually disabled children and second, to acertain the areas of motor performance in which these children differed from normally developing children. As a result of their study Broadhead and Church (1982) claimed that taken together the subtest items of ball throw, standing balance, agility run and drawing a circle accounted for 69.75% of the variance between normal and intellectually disabled children.

Finally, a study by Connolly and Michael (1986) examined differences between intellectually disabled children (IQ range 42–66, mean = 56.8; n=12, age range 7 years 7 months to 10 years 6 months, mean = 9 years 2 months), and children with Down syndrome (IQ range 38–69, mean 54.5: age range 7 years 11 months to 11 years, mean = 9 years 3 months). Scores on the full version of the BOT were used to compare and contrast the motor performance of the two groups of children. The results showed that intellectually disabled children without Down syndrome were significantly better in items measuring running speed and agility, balance, strength, visual–motor control in gross motor skills, and in their fine motor composite scores.

Connolly and Michael (1986) found no significant differences between intellectually disabled boys with and without Down syndrome on the scores for individual subtests. There were, however, significant differences between the scores for girls in the two groups. Girls with Down syndrome had significantly lower scores than their non-Down syndrome intellectually disabled peers, on items measuring running speed, balance, strength, visual motor control and upper limb speed and dexterity. For this reason they claimed that the difference between the two groups of children was mainly due to the lower performance of the girls with Down syndrome. No significant interaction was reported, however, to support their claim of poorer performance in girls with Down syndrome. In addition, there was no significant difference between boys and girls with moderate intellectual disability and Down syndrome, collectively on BOT subtests of bilateral coordination, response time, upper limb speed and dexterity. Connolly and Michael (1986) suggested that the characteristic low muscle tone of children with Down syndrome may have contributed to their lower scores in running and strength items.

In conclusion, the studies reported in this section have shown that both the full version of the BOT and the BOT-S discriminate between the motor performance of normally developing children, and children with motor dysfunction, learning disabilities, mild to moderate intellectual disability and Down syndrome. The fact that both versions of the test tend to place students in a similar ranking within a group has also been confirmed on normally developing children. All the studies have extended some aspect of Bruininks (1978) original data. These results have also demonstrated that the BOT and the BOT-S are valid measures of motor performance, which can be used to determine whether motor impaired children are delayed or different in their motor development, in comparison with normally developing children.

METHOD, RESULTS AND PROCEDURES OF MOTOR PERFORMANCE STUDY

A 2 × 3 factorial design was used. The levels of the two independent variables were as follows. The first factor, age, had two levels, 6 and 10 year olds who were designated younger and older, and was a between-subjects factor. The second factor, category, had three levels, clumsy, intellectually disabled and Down syndrome, and was a between-subjects factor (Table A.1).

Table A.1 Children's age and category groups

Category	*Clumsy children*		*Intellectually disabled*		*Down syndrome*	
Age groups	6	10	6	10	6	10
Age range (years)						
from	4.2	7.11	4.7	7.4	4.2	7.5
to	7.8	11.10	8.4	11.0	7.8	11.11
Mean (years)	5.10	9.8	6.2	10.1	6.0	9.8
Number/gender	8(Boys)	6(Girls)	7(Boys)	5(Girls)	6(Boys)	5(Girls)

Gender/number per category for early and middle childhood

The children in the clumsy category had been referred by teachers, guidance officers, medical practitioners and parents for assessment at the Child Motor Performance Centre (CMPC), and if necessary, to be included in an adapted physical activity programme. They were accompanied by a parent and sometimes by their teacher. On arrival they were included in an ongoing activity session with other children for at least half an hour before they were tested. This served a twofold purpose, first to familiarize the children with the setting and the other children, and second to enable the author to observe and get to know the children before they were tested.

The children with intellectual disability and Down syndrome were part of a school group and so were accompanied by their teachers and sometimes a parent. A similar procedure was followed with these children as the one with the clumsy children, before they were tested.

Children with major physical abnormalities, such as cerebral palsy, or with medical problems which would reduce their physical functioning were not included in the study. The children in all the groups were tested by one examiner, and in the majority of cases the children were with familiar peers.

Procedure

The procedure for the Bruininks–Oseretsky Test (as outlined in the Test Manual; Bruininks, 1978), was used for the items comprising the gross motor component. Scoring was also as presented in the Test Manual. All children were tested individually (but other children were present), on the eight items of the five subtests chosen from the BOT-S. The reported notation of the items is derived from the Examiners Manual, Bruininks–Oseretsky Test of Motor Proficiency (Bruininks, 1978). Performance on all items was assessed on a flat playground surface or a gymnasium surface. Each item was explained verbally and demonstrated by the examiner, then the child performed the item until the examiner thought the child understood what had to be performed. This procedure was essential with some of the younger and some of the intellectually disabled children.

Results

The results are presented for the total raw score on the five items and for each individual item for all the children. The means and standard deviations for the total raw scores on the first five subtests in the Short Form of the Bruininks–Oseretsky Test are shown in Table A.2

An ANOVA conducted on these data indicated that there was an age by category interaction, $F(2, 68) = 5.69$, $P < 0.005$, and main effects for age, $F(1, 68) = 71.85$, $P < 0.01$, and for category, $F(2, 68) = 8.07$, $P < 0.01$. The age by category interaction indicated differences in the overall pattern of performance within the different categories and age groups of children.

Table A.2 Total scores on the adapted version of the Bruininks–Oseretsky Test, Short Form, for children who are clumsy, intellectually disabled and with Down syndrome

Category	*Age group*	*Mean*	*SD*
Clumsy children	6	11.50	4.75
	10	27.29	4.12
Intellectually disabled	6	12.83	6.53
	10	18.75	6.06
Down syndrome	6	8.73	4.84
	10	17.90	5.94

A Newman–Keuls *post hoc* analysis revealed that older clumsy children gained significantly higher scores than moderately intellectually disabled and Down syndrome peers ($P < 0.01$), who did not differ significantly from each other. Further, none of the younger groups differed from each other, but each of the older groups (clumsy, intellectually disabled and Down syndrome) were significantly better than the younger children in the same category ($P < 0.01$). The main effect for age, however, showed that within each category the older age group gained a significantly higher score than the younger group.

Subtest 1/item 1: Running Speed and Agility
(measures running speed during a shuttle run)

An ANOVA on these data showed a main effect for age, $F(1, 68) = 30.93$, $P < 0.001$), and for category, $F(2, 68) = 3.82$, $P < 0.026$, with no age by category interaction. The younger group was significantly slower than the older group across all categories of motor impairment. *Post hoc* analysis of the category main effect indicated that clumsy children were significantly faster than the children with Down syndrome. A summary of the means and standard deviations for the groups is presented in Table A.3.

Table A.3 Scores obtained by children who are clumsy, intellectually disabled and with Down syndrome for running speed and agility: subtest 1/item 1

Category	*Age group*	*Mean*	*SD*
Clumsy children	6	3.64	2.02
	10	7.14	2.21
Intellectually disabled	6	3.83	2.44
	10	5.67	2.17
Down syndrome	6	1.81	2.00
	10	5.36	2.94

Subtest 2/item 2: Static Balance
(standing on preferred leg on balance beam)

The means and standard deviations for this measure are presented in Table A.4. There was an age by category interaction,

Table A.4 Scores obtained by children who are clumsy, intellectually disabled and with Down syndrome for Static Balance: subtest 2/item 2

Category	*Age group*	*Mean*	*SD*
Clumsy children	6	1.00	0.96
	10	3.78	1.85
Intellectually disabled	6	1.25	0.96
	10	1.92	1.08
Down syndrome	6	1.18	0.98
	10	1.54	1.21

$F(2, 68) = 7.09$, $P < 0.002$, and a main effect for age, $F(1, 68) = 23.01$, $P < 0.001$, and for category, $F(2, 68) = 4.95$, $P < 0.01$. Table A.4 shows that the younger group in all categories maintain static balance for a shorter period than the older group. A Newman–Keuls *post hoc* analysis indicated, however, that the older clumsy group maintained balance for a significantly longer time than the older intellectually disabled and Down syndrome groups ($P < 0.01$). Conversely, the younger clumsy group maintained balance for a significantly shorter time than the intellectually disabled or the Down syndrome group ($P < 0.01$).

Subtest 2/item 7: Dynamic Balance (walking forward heel-to-toe on balance beam)

An ANOVA of these data revealed that there was a category by age interaction, $F(2, 68) = 4.62$, $P < 0.01$, and a main effect for age, $F(1, 68) = 16.15$, $P < 0.001$. It should be noted that there was no significant category main effect for this test item. A *post hoc* analysis (Newman–Keuls) of the category by age interaction indicated that the younger clumsy children did not differ significantly from the older intellectually disabled and Down syndrome groups. There was a significant difference, however, between the older clumsy group and the older Down syndrome groups ($P < 0.01$), and the older intellectually disabled group ($P < 0.05$). An

Table A.5 Scores obtained by children who are clumsy, intellectually disabled and with Down syndrome for Dynamic Balance: subtest 2/item 7

Category	*Age group*	*Mean*	*SD*
Clumsy children	6	0.57	0.09
	10	2.42	1.22
Intellectually disabled	6	1.17	0.97
	10	1.50	1.09
Down syndrome	6	0.93	0.70
	10	1.54	0.97

inspection of the means and standard deviations for the groups (Table A.5), shows the age by category interaction.

Subtest 3/item 1: Bilateral coordination (tapping feet alternately while making circles with fingers)

This item was scored on a pass or fail basis, so no means are available. It should be noted that very few children were able to pass this item in the 10-year-old clumsy group, and none of the other motor impaired children passed this item.

Subtest 3/item 6: Bilateral Coordination (jumping up and clapping hands)

The ANOVA revealed that there was a significant age by category interaction, $F(2, 68) = 5.15$, $P < 0.01$, a main effect for age, $F(1, 68) = 21.20$, $P < 0.001$ and for category, $F(2, 68) = 6.70$

Table A.6 Scores obtained by clumsy children, intellectually disabled and Down syndrome children for jump and clap hands: subtest 3/item 6

Category	*Age group*	*Mean*	*SD*
Clumsy children	6	1.00	0.78
	10	2.57	1.02
Intellectually disabled	6	0.92	0.67
	10	1.17	0.58
Down syndrome	6	0.91	0.83
	10	1.45	0.91

$P < 0.003$. The means and standard deviations are presented in Table A.6.

The Newman–Keuls *post hoc* analysis for the age by category interaction showed that the children in the older clumsy group were significantly better coordinated than children in all of the other age and category groups ($P < 0.01$). As in the two balance items, the significant difference for category was due to the better performance of the older clumsy children, who scored higher on this test item than any other group.

Subtest 4/item 1: strength (standing broad jump)

In the ANOVA for this item there was an age by category interaction, $F(2, 68) = 3.22$, $P < 0.045$, a main effect for age, $F(1, 68) = 65.37$, $P < 0.01$, and for category, $F(2, 68) = 3.90$, $P < 0.024$.

The *post hoc* analysis (Newman–Keuls) for the age by category interaction showed that the younger groups of clumsy, intellectually disabled and Down syndrome children scored significantly lower than the older clumsy group ($P < 0.01$). Also, children in the older clumsy group scored significantly higher than the older intellectually disabled and Down syndrome groups ($P < 0.05$). In addition, older intellectually disabled and Down syndrome groups scored significantly higher than the younger clumsy and children with Down syndrome ($P < 0.01$). The *post hoc* analysis for category revealed that clumsy children scored significantly higher than children with Down sydrome, but did not differ significantly from the intellectually disabled children ($P < 0.05$), (Table A.7).

Table A.7 Scores obtained by children who are clumsy, intellectually disabled and with Down syndrome for standing broad jump. subtest 4/item 4

Category	*Age group*	*Mean*	*SD*
Clumsy children	6	3.00	1.47
	10	7.21	1.19
Intellectually disabled	6	3.41	2.02
	10	5.33	2.06
Down syndrome	6	2.36	1.21
	10	5.27	1.74

Subtest 5/item 3: upper limb coordination
(catching a tossed ball with both hands)

An ANOVA on these data revealed a main effect for age, $F\ (1, 68) = 15.32$, $P < 0.01$ and category $F(2, 68) = 3.96$, $P < 0.023$ with no interactions. The means and standard deviations are presented in Table A.8. The analysis indicated that the children in the older groups scored significantly higher than the younger age groups. A *post hoc* analysis (Newman–Keuls) of the category main effect indicated that the clumsy children were significantly better coordinated than the Down syndrome group ($P < 0.01$), and the intellectually disabled group ($P < 0.05$).

Table A.8 Scores obtained by children who are clumsy, intellectually disabled and with Down syndrome for catching a tossed ball: subtest 5/item 3

Category	*Age group*	*Mean*	*SD*
Clumsy children	6	1.14	1.03
	10	2.28	0.82
Intellectually disabled	6	1.17	0.71
	10	1.67	1.07
Down syndrome	6	0.64	0.67
	10	1.36	0.92

Subtest 5/item 5: upper limb coordination
(throwing a ball at a target with preferred hand)

The ANOVA for these data revealed a main effect for age,

Table A.9 Scores obtained by children who are clumsy, intellectually disabled and with Down syndrome for throwing: subtest 5/item 5

Category	*Age group*	*Mean*	*SD*
Clumsy children	6	1.00	0.68
	10	2.07	1.64
Intellectually disabled	6	0.75	0.62
	10	1.33	0.77
Down syndrome	6	0.90	0.70
	10	1.27	0.79

$F(1, 68) = 9.870$, $P < 0.003$. This item only distinguished then between the younger group of children who scored significantly lower than the older children. The means and standard deviations are presented in Table A.9.

REFERENCES

Broadhead, G.D. and Bruininks, R.H. (1982) Childhood motor performance traits on the Short Form Bruininks–Oseretsky Test. *Special Populations*, Oct., 149–55.

Broadhead, G.D. and Bruininks, R.H. (1983a) Development of motor proficiency factors throughout childhood. *Physical Educator*, **40**, 16–19.

Broadhead, G.D. and Bruininks, R.H. (1983b) Factor structure consistency in the Bruininks–Oseretsky Test Short Form. *Rehabilitation Literature*, **44**, 13–18.

Bruininks, R. (1978) Bruininks–Oseretsky Test of Motor Proficiency: Examiners Manual. Minnesota American Guidance Service, Centre Pines, MN.

Bruininks, V.L. and Bruininks, R.H. (1977) Motor proficiency of learning disabled and nondisabled students. *Perceptual and Motor Skills*, **44**, 1131–7.

Connolly, B.H. and Michael, B.T. (1986) Performance of retarded children with and without Down's Syndrome, on the Bruininks-Oseretsky Test of Motor Proficiency. *Physical Therapy*, **66**, 344–8.

Haubenstricker, J., Seefeldt, V., Fountain, C. and Sapp, M. (1981) The efficiency of the Bruininks-Oseretsky Test of Motor Proficiency in discriminating between normal children and those with gross motor dysfunction. Paper presented at the Pre-Convention Symposium of the Motor Development Academy, National Association for Sport and Physical Education, Boston.

Kirk, S.A. and Gallagher, J.J. (1986) *Educating Exceptional Children*. Houghton Mifflin, Boston.

Krus, P.H., Bruininks, R.H. and Robertson, G. (1981) Structure of motor abilities in children. *Perceptual and Motor Skills*, **52**, 119–29.

Roswal, G.M. (1983) Developmental play program on the motor proficiency of mildly handicapped children. *American Corrective Therapy Journal*, **37**, 105–8.

Appendix B
Fundamental movement patterns

METHOD

Four different categories of children participated in this study. These were normally developing children (designated normal) who attended state preschools and primary schools in the Brisbane Region, and children who are clumsy, intellectually disabled or have Down syndrome. (See Appendix A for more details about the motor impaired children selected for the studies.)

The design consisted of a 2 × 4 factorial design. The levels of the two independent variables were as follows: age, two levels, younger and older; and category which comprised children who are normal, clumsy, intellectually disabled or have Down syndrome. Table B.1 presents the age ranges, mean age and numbers of children in each group.

PROCEDURE

All subjects were assessed individually by the author, either in a large flat open area such as an oval or playground, or in the gymnasium of the Department of Human Movement Studies at the University of Queensland. Each subject was told that the assessor was looking at how well he or she could walk, run, jump, catch and throw. For the walking and running conditions, subjects were observed from behind, side-on and from the front, while they walked or ran as fast as possible, continuously backwards and forwards for 25 metres, in a straight

Table B.1 Children's age and category groups

Category and age	*Mean (years, months)*	*Age range*		*Number*
		From	*To*	
Normal				
6 years	5.1	4.3	7.4	15
10 years	10.5	8.8	11.11	15
Clumsy				
6 years	5.4	4.3	7.4	15
10 years	9.7	7.8	11.11	15
Intellectually disabled				
6 years	5.8	4.8	7.2	14
10 years	9.8	8.1	11.10	15
Down syndrome				
6 years	5.2	4.2	7.2	14
10 years	10.00	8.1	11.10	14

line on a flat surface. The jumping condition consisted of asking the subject to perform a standing broad jump from behind a marked line. The subject was required to place both feet on this line and was then told to perform a single two leg jump 'as far as you can'. This task was repeated three times. In the catching condition the subjects were positioned facing a blank wall so they were not distracted by other children. The examiner observed from the side and front, while another person faced the subject and threw a ball, five times, at a moderate speed from 2–5 metres away (depending on the age of the subject). A tennis ball was used for the older groups and a soft sponge ball (nerf ball), of the same size as a tennis ball, was thrown to the younger children. In order to assess the child's throwing pattern, the examiner observed the child from the front, back and the side, as the child threw the ball 'as far as possible' (five times). To obtain a total fundamental movement pattern score and total walking, running, jumping, catching and throwing score, the examiner marked off the observational level for an individual, in each of the elements that comprised a particular movement profile for each subject. The check-list observations were converted into a score by giving 1 point for each element of the pattern at level 1, 2 points for each element of the pattern at level 2, 3 points for each element of the pattern at level 3, and 4 points for each level of the pattern at level 4. This scoring system enabled the fundamental movement patterns for each age group and category of children to be compared, in terms of a total fundamental movement pattern score and in terms of total scores for each of the movement patterns and for the elements in each pattern.

RESULTS AND DISCUSSION

The analyses of the total fundamental movement patterns (FMP) scores, the walking, running, jumping, catching and throwing scores and the element scores for each individual movement pattern revealed a main effect for age. Irrespective of the children's category the younger groups of children had less mature movement pattern scores than the older groups of children.

The results obtained from each of the analyses will be discussed under the following headings: total fundamental pattern scores; walking, running, jumping, catching and throwing scores.

Total fundamental movement pattern (FMP) scores

For this analysis the score for each of the elements within each movement profile were added to give a total FMP score. Tables B.2 and B.3 give the category and for age means, SDs and F values, respectively.

A Newman–Keuls *post hoc* analysis for category showed that the normal group were significantly more mature in their total FMP scores than the children who are clumsy, intellectually

Table B.2 Means (SDs) and F values of total fundamental movement pattern scores for normal, clumsy, intellectually disabled and Down syndrome groups

	Normal	*Clumsy*	*Intellectually disabled*	*Down syndrome*	*F (df)*
Total scores FMP	72.82 (12.71)	59.50 (12.78)	51.57 (13.78)	43.37 (15.65)	$F(3, 116) = 55.30$ ($P<0.001$)

able B.3 Means (SDs) and *F* values of total fundamental movement pattern scores for younger (6 year old) and older (10 year old) children

	Age group		
	6	*10*	F *(df)*
Total scores FMP	47.16 (11.73)	68.53 (14.52)	*F*(1, 116) = 184.63 (*P*<0.001)

disabled or have Down syndrome (*P*<0.01). The clumsy group of children were also significantly more mature than the intellectually disabled and Down syndrome groups, who did not significantly differ from each other, even though there was a trend for lower scores in the Down syndrome group.

Walking

The results of the ANOVA are reported in Tables B.4 and B.5 and the Newman–Keuls *post hoc* results for category are reported in Table B.6.

The main effect for age indicated that the younger children had a less mature walking pattern than the older children, for the total walking pattern. This trend was also evident in all the elements that comprise the walking pattern in both normal and motor impaired children.

The *post hoc* analysis revealed that the significant difference between the categories was because the normal children had a more mature pattern in total walking than the clumsy children who had a more mature total pattern than the other motor impaired children (Table B.6).

The results reported in Table B.6 also indicate that clumsy children were at a more mature level in their general body appearance, in transfer of weight, symmetry of leg action and stride length. In fact it was these latter aspects related to lower limb action that showed a significant difference between each group, with normal children exhibiting a more mature pattern than the intellectually disabled and Down syndrome groups, respectively. In contrast, the action of the upper body and limbs only distinguished between the normal children and motor impaired children as a group as they did not differ from each other.

Table B.4 Means (SDs) and *F* values for total walking score and element walking scores of clumsy, intellectually disabled and Down syndrome groups

	Normal	*Clumsy*	*Intellectually disabled*	*Down syndrome*	F *(d/f)*
Total score walking	16.64 (2.69)	13.03 (3.32)	11.43 (2.50)	10.00 (2.27)	$F(3, 116) = 62.80$ ($P<0.001$)
General body appearance	3.21 (0.56)	2.57 (0.82)	2.42 (0.72)	2.03 (0.56)	$F(3, 116) = 24.48$ ($P<0.001$)
Upper body and limbs	3.27 (0.63)	2.66 (0.71)	2.58 (0.67)	2.30 (0.70)	$F(3, 116) = 16.16$ ($P<0.001$)
Lower body and limbs	3.37 (0.60)	2.57 (0.68)	2.23 (0.58)	1.97 (0.55)	$F(3, 116) = 44.24$ ($P<0.001$)
Basis of movement pattern	3.34 (0.61)	2.73 (0.64)	2.19 (0.70)	1.80 (0.16)	$F(3, 116) = 61.46$ ($P<0.001$)
Additional criteria	3.40 (0.61)	2.50 (0.86)	2.26 (0.58)	1.90 (0.66)	$F(3, 116) = 42.29$ ($P<0.001$)

Table B.5 Means (SDs) and *F* values for total walking score and element walking scores for each age group

	Age groups		
	6	*10*	F *(df)*
Total score Walking	11.08 (2.80)	14.63 (3.63)	$F(1, 116) = 93.69$ ($P<0.001$)
General body appearance	2.23 (0.64)	2.92 (0.77)	$F(1, 116) = 47.$[illegible]1 ($P<0.001$)
Upper body and limbs	2.35 (0.65)	3.08 (0.68)	$F(1, 116) = 49.29$ ($P<0.001$)
Lower body and limbs	2.24 (0.62)	2.89 (0.[illegible]3)	$F(1, 116) = 50.19$ ($P<0.001$)
Basis of movement pattern	2.15 (0.67)	2.95 (0.88)	$F(1, 116) = 82.02$ ($P<0.001$)
Additional criteria	2.13 (0.69)	2.94 (0.87)	$F(1, 116) = 65.82$ ($P<0.001$)

Table B.6 Results of Newman–Keuls *post hoc* analyses for total walking score and element walking scores for each category

Total walking score
Normal** > Clumsy**> Intellectually disabled = Down syndrome

General body appearance[a]
Normal**> Clumsy**> Intellectually disabled** > Down syndrome

Upper body and limbs
Normal** > Clumsy = Intellectually disabled = Down syndrome

Lower body and limbs[a]
Normal** > Clumsy** > Intellectually disabled* > Down syndrome

Basis of movement pattern
Normal* > Clumsy** > Intellectually disabled = Down syndrome

Additional criteria
Normal* > Clumsy** > Intellectually disabled = Down syndrome

*$P<0.05$; **$P<0.01$ ***$P<0.001$.

[a]Element discriminated between each category.

Running

Tables B.7, B.8 and B.9 summarize the results of the analyses for the running pattern.

Table B.7 Means (SDs) and *F* values for total running score and element running scores of clumsy, intellectually disabled and Down syndrome groups

	Normal	*Clumsy*	*Intellectually disabled*	*Down syndrome*	F *(d/f)*
Total score running	15.79 (2.50)	12.30 (3.15)	10.80 (2.71)	9.80 (2.90)	$F(3, 116) = 52.00$ ($P<0.001$)
General body appearance	3.39 (0.61)	2.50 (0.86)	2.26 (0.58)	1.90 (0.66)	$F(3, 116) = 42.29$ ($P<0.001$)
Upper body and limbs	3.18 (0.63)	2.50 (0.82)	2.30 (0.69)	2.50 (0.68)	$F(3, 116) = 11.61$ ($P<0.001$)
Lower body and limbs	3.12 (0.49)	2.37 (0.56)	2.16 (0.68)	1.77 (0.68)	$F(3, 116) = 40.04$ ($P<0.001$)
Basis of movement pattern	3.09 (0.58)	2.43 (0.68)	2.16 (0.64)	1.80 (0.76)	$F(3, 116) = 31.98$ ($P<0.001$)
Additional criteria	3.27 (0.72)	2.53 (0.73)	2.23 (0.72)	1.83 (0.59)	$F(3, 116) = 42.34$ ($P<0.001$)

Table B.8 Means (SDs) and *F* values for total running score and element running scores for each age group

	Age groups		
	6	*10*	F *(df)*
Total score Running	10.33 (3.00)	14.06 (3.16)	$F(1, 116) = 107.40$ ($P<0.001$)
General body appearance	2.13 (0.69)	2.94 (0.87)	$F(1, 116) = 65.82$ ($P<0.001$)
Upper body and limbs	2.19 (0.74)	3.06 (0.70)	$F(1, 116) = 55.95$ ($P<0.001$)
Lower body and limbs	2.03 (0.68)	2.71 (0.73)	$F(1, 116) = 55.32$ ($P<0.001$)
Basis of movement pattern	2.00 (0.73)	2.77 (0.70)	$F(1, 116) = 62.93$ ($P<0.001$)
Additional criteria	2.03 (0.70)	2.94 (0.79)	$F(1, 116) = 90.83$ ($P<0.001$)

Table B.9 Results of Newman–Keuls *post hoc* analyses for total running score and element running scores for each category

Total running score
  Normal = Clumsy** > Intellectually disabled = Down syndrome

General body appearance
  Normal*> Clumsy = Intellectually disabled* > Down syndrome

Upper body and limbs
  Normal** > Clumsy = Intellectually disabled = Down syndrome

Lower body and limbs[a]
  Normal** > Clumsy** > Intellectually disabled* > Down syndrome

Basis of movement pattern
  Normal** > Clumsy** > Intellectually disabled = Down syndrome

Additional criteria
  Normal** > Clumsy** > Intellectually disabled = Down syndrome

*$P<0.05$; **$P<0.01$; ***$P<0.001$.

[a]Element discriminated between each category.

The results of the running pattern are similar to the walking pattern since the younger children's total running pattern and all its elements were significantly less mature than the older children. Furthermore, normal children were significantly more mature than the children who are intellectually disabled or have Down syndrome but not their clumsy peers.

In general body appearance, normal children were significantly more mature than the clumsy children. Results for the upper body and limb action only distinguished between the normal and clumsy, but not between the intellectually disabled and Down syndrome groups. In contrast the lower body and limb action distinguished between each of the four groups of children. Clumsy children when compared with their motor impaired peers were significantly more mature than children with Down syndrome in the elements of general body appearance, basis of the movement pattern and additional criteria. Their running pattern was not more mature than the intellectually disabled children in general body appearance, upper body and limb action and the basis of the movement pattern. Clumsy children, however, were more mature than intellectually disabled children in their lower limb action in terms of a more powerful leg action and length of stride.

Jumping

The analyses of the total jumping and element jumping scores are reported in Tables B.10, B.11 and B.12.

In the jumping pattern the main effects for age and category were significant. The levels attained for each age for children in the different categories were also similar to the walking and running patterns (Table B.12).

The results for the analyses of the total jumping score, general body appearance, upper body and limbs, lower body and limbs, basis of the movement pattern and the additional criteria revealed that normal children were significantly more mature than the motor impaired groups. In addition, clumsy children were significantly more mature in total jumping score and all the elements than the intellectually disabled and Down syndrome group who did not differ from each other. In the jumping pattern, therefore, all the analyses distinguished between the normal and clumsy children but not between children who are intellectually disabled or have Down syndrome.

Table B.10 Means (SDs) and *F* values for total jumping score and element jumping scores of clumsy, intellectually disabled and Down syndrome groups

	Normal	*Clumsy*	*Intellectually disabled*	*Down syndrome*	F *(df)*
Total score jumping	14.36 (2.16)	12.10 (2.37)	9.30 (2.83)	9.13 (3.46)	$F(3, 116) = 37.70$ ($P<0.001$)
General body appearance	2.81 (0.58)	2.47 (0.51)	2.00 (0.58)	1.93 (0.58)	$F(3, 116) = 22.35$ ($P<0.001$)
Upper body and limbs	2.90 (0.46)	2.53 (0.51)	2.03 (0.80)	1.77 (0.90)	$F(3, 116) = 23.81$ ($P<0.001$)
Lower body and limbs	2.88 (0.54)	2.40 (0.50)	1.77 (0.67)	1.77 (0.77)	$F(3, 116) = 30.04$ ($P<0.001$)
Basis of movement pattern	2.94 (0.50)	2.33 (0.66)	1.81 (0.65)	1.90 (0.76)	$F(3, 116) = 26.04$ ($P<0.001$)
Additional criteria	2.81 (0.64)	2.37 (0.49)	1.87 (0.72)	1.77 (0.82)	$F(3, 116) = 1.78$ ($P<0.001$)

Table B.11 Means (SDs) and *F* values for total jumping score and element jumping scores for each age group

	Age group		
	6	*10*	F *(df)*
Total score jumping	9.75 (3.05)	12.82 (3.22)	$F(1, 116) = 5.53$ ($P<0.001$)
General body appearance	2.03 (0.60)	2.60 (0.61)	$F(1, 116) = 40.16$ ($P<0.001$)
Upper body and limbs	2.00 (0.79)	2.68 (0.67)	$F(1, 116) = 45.41$ ($P<0.001$)
Lower body and limbs	1.92 (0.73)	2.52 (0.72)	$F(1, 116) = 36.03$ ($P<0.001$)
Basis of movement pattern	1.95 (0.73)	2.56 (0.71)	$F(1, 116) = 35.46$ ($P<0.001$)
Additional criteria	1.87 (0.66)	2.56 (0.76)	$F(1, 116) = 43.50$ ($P<0.001$)

Table B.12 Results of Newman–Keuls *post hoc* analyses for total jumping score and element jumping scores for each category

Total jumping score	
	Normal** > Clumsy**> Intellectually disabled = Down syndrome
General body appearance	
	Normal* > Clumsy* > Intellectually disabled = Down syndrome
Upper body and limbs	
	Normal** > Clumsy** > Intellectually disabled = Down syndrome
Lower body and limbs	
	Normal** > Clumsy** > Intellectually disabled = Down syndrome
Basis of movement pattern	
	Normal** > Clumsy** > Intellectually disabled = Down syndrome
Additional criteria	
	Normal** > Clumsy** > Intellectually disabled = Down syndrome

*$P<0.05$; **$P<0.01$; ***$P<0.001$.

Catching

The analyses for the catching pattern are summarized in Tables B.13, B.14 and B.15.

Once again main effects for age and category were significant. The younger children were less mature in their total catching pattern. Normal children also had a more mature catching pattern than motor impaired children in their total movement pattern as well as most of the elements. An exception was the additional criteria element in which normal and clumsy children were similar.

General body appearance was the element which distinguished between all categories, with normal children having a significantly more mature pattern, than clumsy children who were significantly more mature than the intellectually disabled and Down syndrome groups, respectively. The lower body and limb pattern in catching did not distinguish between the motor impaired groups, in contrast to the walking and running patterns where it distinguished between all the groups. It should be noted that although the catching levels were lower than those for the locomotor patterns, they were similar to the levels attained in the throwing pattern which are reported in the next section.

Table B.13 Means (SDs) and *F* values for total catching score and element catching scores of clumsy, intellectually disabled and Down syndrome groups

	Normal	*Clumsy*	*Intellec-tually disabled*	*Down syn-drome*	F*(d/f)*
Total score catching	13.24 (3.42)	10.83 (3.81)	9.27 (3.32)	8.47 (4.16)	*F*(3, 116) = 23.29 (*P*<0.001)
General body appearance	2.67 (0.74)	2.27 (0.94)	1.97 (0.66)	1.70 (0.80)	*F*(3, 116) = 17.70 (*P*<0.001)
Upper body and limbs	2.64 (0.74)	2.17 (0.83)	1.98 (0.73)	1.70 (0.87)	*F*(3, 116) = 15.14 (*P*<0.001)
Lower body and limbs	2.61 (0.83)	2.07 (0.69)	1.84 (0.74)	1.67 (0.84)	*F*(3, 116) = 16.73 (*P*<0.001)
Basis of move-ment pattern	2.76 (0.75)	2.20 (0.76)	1.77 (0.76)	1.66 (0.92)	*F*(3, 116) = 22.70 (*P*<0.001)
Additional criteria	2.61 (0.70)	2.13 (0.82)	1.90 (0.75)	1.73 (0.87)	*F*(3, 116) = 15.04 (*P*<0.001)

Table B.14 Means (SDs) and *F* values for total catching score and element catching scores for each age group

	Age groups		
	6	*10*	F*(df)*
Total score catching	7.75 (2.62)	13.24 (3.39)	*F*(1, 116) = 153.60 (*P*<0.001)
General body appearance	1.61 (0.55)	2.71 (0.76)	*F*(1, 116) = 121.46 (*P*<0.001)
Upper body and limbs	1.56 (0.75)	2.66 (0.60)	*F*(1, 116) = 108.54 (*P*<0.001)
Lower body and limbs	1.52 (0.56)	[illegible] (0.70)	*F*(1, 116) = 113.54 (*P*<0.001)
Basis of move-ment pattern	1.55 (0.56)	2.66 (0.70)	*F*(1, 116) = 126.28 (*P*<0.001)
Additional criteria	1.56 (0.60)	2.66 (0.81)	*F*(1, 116) = 108.19 (*P*<0.001)

Table B.15 Results of Newman–Keuls *post hoc* analyses for total catching score and element catching scores for each category

Total catching score
Normal* > Clumsy*> Intellectually disabled = Down syndrome
General body appearance[a]
Normal** > Clumsy** > Intellectually disabled* > Down syndrome
Upper body and limbs
Normal** > Clumsy** > = Intellectually disabled = Down syndrome
Lower body and limbs
Normal** > Clumsy = Intellectually disabled = Down syndrome
Basis of movement pattern
Normal** > Clumsy = Intellectually disabled* = Down syndrome
Additional criteria
Normal = Clumsy** > Intellectually disabled = Down syndrome

[a]Element discriminated between each category. *$P<0.05$; **$P<0.01$; ***$P<0.001$.

Throwing

The analyses for throwing are summarized in Tables B.16, B.17 and B.18.

The analyses for throwing revealed main effects for age and category as was found in the other FMPs. This movement pattern, however, differed from the walking, running and catching results, but not the jumping, in that not one of the elements distinguished between all the groups of children.

Table B.18 reveals that normal children were similar to clumsy children in terms of their total throwing pattern and in the elements of general body appearance, upper body and limbs, lower body and limbs and the basis of the movement pattern. In general body appearance, upper body and limbs and additional criteria, there was no significant difference between the normal, clumsy and intellectually disabled children, though these three groups were significantly more mature than the Down syndrome group. (See Appendix A.)

The throwing and element throwing scores generally only distinguished between the normal and Down syndrome groups of children, but not between clumsy, intellectually disabled and Down syndrome groups. Moreover, the developmental levels reached by each group were lower than the level they had achieved in the locomotor patterns, but similar to their level in their catching pattern.

Table B.16 Means (SDs) and F values for total throwing score and element throwing scores of clumsy, intellectually disabled and Down syndrome groups

	Normal	*Clumsy*	*Intellectually disabled*	*Down syndrome*	F *(df)*
Total score walking	12.80 (4.16)	11.20 (3.58)	10.00 (4.21)	9.07 (4.60)	$F(3, 116) = 7.71$ ($P<0.001$)
General body appearance	2.55 (0.83)	2.27 (0.87)	2.00 (0.86)	1.80 (0.89)	$F(3, 116) = 6.72$ ($P<0.001$)
Upper body and limbs	2.48 (0.80)	2.17 (0.75)	2.00 (0.91)	1.73 (0.94)	$F(3, 116) = 5.84$ ($P<0.001$)
Lower body and limbs	2.48 (0.83)	2.27 (0.82)	2.03 (0.88)	1.87 (0.97)	$F(3, 116) = 4.16$ ($P<0.01$)
Basis of movement pattern	2.52 (1.00)	2.23 (0.73)	2.00 (0.90)	1.83 (1.10)	$F(3, 116) = 5.03$ ($P<0.003$)
Additional criteria	2.76 (1.03)	2.27 (0.78)	2.13 (0.92)	1.93 (1.11)	$F(3, 116) = 6.78$ ($P<0.001$)

Table B.17 Means (SDs) and F values for total throwing score and element throwing scores for each age group

	Age groups		
	6	*10*	F *(df)*
Total score throwing	8.21 (3.29)	13.37 (3.70)	$F(1, 116) = 77.39$ ($P<0.001$)
General body appearance	1.66 (0.72)	2.50 (0.77)	$F(1, 116) = 62.96$ ($P<0.001$)
Upper body and limbs	1.66 (0.70)	2.60 (0.80)	$F(1, 116) = 53.12$ ($P<0.001$)
Lower body and limbs	1.69 (0.74)	2.65 (0.79)	$F(1, 116) = 50.74$ ($P<0.001$)
Basis of movement pattern	1.61 (0.86)	2.70 (0.69)	$F(1, 116) = 65.83$ ($P<0.001$)
Additional criteria	1.10 (0.70)	2.87 (0.93)	$F(1, 116) = 73.78$ ($P<0.001$)

Table B.16 Results of Newman–Keuls *post hoc* analyses for total throwing score and element throwing scores for each category

Total throwing score	Normal = Clumsy** > Intellectually disabled = Down syndrome
General body appearance	Normal = Clumsy = Intellectually disabled** > Down syndrome
Upper body and limbs	Normal = Clumsy = Intellectually disabled** > Down syndrome
Lower body and limbs	Normal = Clumsy = Intellectually disabled** > Down syndrome
Basis of movement pattern	Normal = Clumsy** > Intellectually disabled* > Down syndrome
Additional criteria	Normal* > Down syndrome Normal = Clumsy = Intellectually disabled

*$P<0.05$; **$P<0.01$; ***$P<0.001$.

Appendix C
The motor control study

METHOD

A total of 64 children participated in this experiment, 48 of whom were new subjects and the data from the 10 and 6 year old grouping (a previous study) were incorporated as a baseline measure of normally developing children's motor control. In this study the children were divided into two age groups (10 and 6 years) and four categories (each with four boys and four girls), as follows. The mean ages were: normally developing children (all of whom attended state primary schools), 6 years 4 months (range 5 years 7 months–7 years 5 months) and 10 years 8 months (range 9 years 7 months–11 years 9 months); clumsy children (all these children attended state primary schools), 6 years 1 month (range 5 years 0 months–7 years 3 months), and 10 years 8 months (range 9 years 7 months–11 years 9 months); intellectually disabled children (who attended state special schools), 6 years 7 months (range 5 years 11 months–7 years 4 months) and 10 years 3 months (range 8 years 11 months–11 years 11 months); Down syndrome children (who attended state schools and state special schools), 6 years 4 months (range 5 years 0 months–7 years 4 months) and 10 years 6 months (range 9 years 6 months–11 years 4 months).

All children who participated in this experiment had parental permission. Children in the clumsy, intellectually disabled, and Down syndrome categories had been referred to the Child Motor Performance Centre at the Department of Human Movement Studies, University of Queensland. These subjects were at least one standard deviation below their age appropriate motor performance levels on the Bruininks–Oseretsky Test of Motor Proficiency (BOT, Chapter 5), and were selected randomly to participate in the study (Appendix A has provided details about the children who participated in the studies reported in this book).

PROCEDURE

A 2 × 4 × 4 × 2 × 2 × 2 factorial design was used in this study. The first factor had two age groups, designated 6 and 10 years. The second factor had four categories of children, normal, clumsy, intellectually disabled and Down syndrome, both these factors were between factor variables. All other factors were within subject variables. These were: the condition factor at four levels (i.e., 10(L):10(R), 30(L):30(R), 10(L):30(R), 30(L):10(R); hands factor (left and right hand); the distance moved by each hand (either 10 cm or 30 cm); and whether both hands moved the same or a different distance (same or different). All results were analysed by ANOVA and the Newman–Keuls procedure. The measurements were response time, movement time, total movement time and spatial accuracy.

RESULTS

Response time analysis

An ANOVA was conducted on the response time data. This revealed main effects for age, $F(1, 56) = 7.82$, $P < 0.007$; for category, $F(3, 56) = 11.14$, $P < 0.001$; for distance $F(1, 56) = 53.34$, $P < .001$; and an interaction for age by category, $F(3, 56) = 3.43$, $P < 0.023$ and for category by distance, $F(3, 56) = 5.77$, $P < 0.002$.

The main effect for age was due to the fact that the 10 year old group had a significantly faster response time (mean 388.66 ms, SD 145.73) than the 6 year old group (mean 473.13, SD 213, 96). The main effect for distance indicated that it took the children a mean response time of 386.58 ms (SD 175.59) before they started moving to the 10 cm target which was significantly faster than when they were required to move to a target 30 cm away (mean 475.21, SD 189.27).

Table C.1 Means and (SDs) for response time (ms) of normal, clumsy, intellectually disabled and Down syndrome groups

Category	*Mean*	*(SD)*
Normal children	315.43	(76.97)
Clumsy children	439.65	(222.35)
Intellectually disabled	559.53	(194.27)
Down syndrome	408.97	(134.04)

A *post hoc* analysis of the category main effect, revealed that intellectually disabled children were significantly slower in response time when compared with normal children, clumsy children and children with Down syndrome ($P < 0.01$). In addition normal children were significantly faster in response time than children who are clumsy or with Down syndrome ($P < 0.05$). The means and standard deviations are shown in Table C.1.

Movement time analysis

Result of the ANOVA for movement time revealed main effects for age, $F(1, 56) = 28.70$, $P < 0.001$, for category, $F(3, 56) = 29.85$, $P < 0.001$, for distance, $F(1, 56) = 11.55$, $P < 0.002$, and age by category interaction, $F(3, 56) = 4.25$, $P < 0.009$, and a category by distance interaction, $F(3, 56) = 5.95$, $P < 0.002$. The ANOVA indicated that 10 year old children had a significantly faster movement time than 6 year olds. The means were 311.48 (SD 119.55) and 428.70 (SD 190.03), respectively. Similarly, when subjects moved 10 cm (collapsed across age, category hand and same/different movement), they were significantly faster than when they moved 30 cm. The means were 353.43 (SD 140.33), for 10 cm and 386.76 (SD 192.48) for 30 cm, respectively.

A *post hoc* analysis of the category main effect revealed that normal and clumsy children did not have significantly different movement times. Down syndrome children, however, had a significantly slower movement time than normal, clumsy and intellectually disabled children ($P < 0.01$). The intellectually disabled children in turn had a significantly slower movement

Table C.2 Mean movement time (ms) and (SDs) for categories

Category	*Mean*	*(SD)*
Normal	253.98	(53.68)
Clumsy	314.79	(100.23)
Intellectually disabled	379.48	(97.03)
Down syndrome	532.12	(222.47)

time than normal children ($P < 0.01$), and also significantly slower than their clumsy age peers ($P < 0.05$) (see Table C.2), for means and standard deviations).

Total movement time analysis

Total movement time is the sum of the two measures (response time and movement time) and represents the total time taken to move the styli from the starting plates to the end plates once the starting beeper was 'set off'. The ANOVA of the total movement time data revealed main effects for age, $F(1, 56) = 28.88$, $P < 0.001$; for category, $F(3, 56)$, $P < 0.001$; for distance, $F(1, 56) = 84.36$, $P < 0.001$; for same and different movement, $F(1, 56) = 4.39$, $P < 0.038$. There were also interactions for same and different movements and left and right hand, $F(1, 56) = 5.16$, $P < 0.025$, and an age by category interaction, $F(3, 56) = 3.87$, $P < 0.014$.

As in the other three measures in this experiment the results of the ANOVA showed that the younger children were significantly slower (mean 909.1444, SD 288.85) than the older age group (mean 701.39, SD 146.95). Also when subjects moved 30 cm they were significantly slower than when they moved 10 cm (the mean total movement times are 746.19, SD 253.91 and 864.34, SD 282.58, respectively). However, unlike the previous ANOVA in this experiment there was a significant difference in total movement time when the hands moved the same distance either 10 cm or 30 cm (mean 790.18, SD 264.29), than when they each moved simultaneously to targets at different distances (i.e. 30(L):106(R) or 10(L):30(R)) where the mean was 820.35 (SD 284.65; $P < 0.01$).